Hold Your Premie

a workbook on skin-to-skin contact
for parents of premature babies

This book is dedicated to our children, Rebecka, Simon and Emma, who give us our greatest joy! My husband and I have both had wonderful parents who gave us love, fun and a secure base of trust to build our lives. We have tried to do the same for our children.

First Published in South Africa 2010
by
New Voices Publishing
Cape Town, South Africa
www.newvoices.co.za

First Edition February 2010 in paperback
Second Edition June 2010
USA Edition November 2010

ISBN: 978-1-920411-33-6 (USA)

DISCLAIMER.

Mother-infant skin-to-skin contact is a safe place to care for newborn and premature
babies – but should only be practiced safely, and under the supervision and
responsibility of health professionals. Authors accept no liability for any adverse
events. The information and advice expressed in this book are believed to be accurate,
and based on the best evidence available. This book is NOT a substitute for current
care in any way; premature newborns should be cared for by health professionals
practicing evidence based medicine.

The publisher is not responsible for errors or omissions.

HOW TO USE THIS BOOK

This is a practical workbook

It has been written to help you Mom and Dad in the scary situation of expecting or having a premature or preterm baby (or just "premie").

It gives <u>key information</u> needed to understand the premie and the NICU (the Neonatal Intensive Care Unit).

It describes <u>practical steps</u> and tasks that help parents be central in the team that is helping their premie.

This book is also a tool for health workers to encourage and empower parents.

<u>To Mom and Dad:</u>

This book is organized into chapters for easy reference. Though they have an order, you can read them in any order you like.

If your premie is already born, then the most important information you will find quickly and easily on the key pages with cross-hatched edges. These are front page summaries of each chapter of what you want to know, and you can start by reading only these.

You will then know where to look for more details, in the pages that follow.

Read the other sections as you need them.

If you are likely to have a premature baby, try to read this book before your baby is born. Understanding the importance of the first hour after birth will help you and your premie.

This is a workbook, so you will see spaces where you can write things down, for example, your own premie's details, treatment, and some of your own reactions. There are suggestions of things to do or observe. You may find this helpful in this difficult time. I encourage you strongly to read through the chapter on "Emotions". Seeing these things written down will help you face them. This is important for you to cope better for yourself and so be better able to help your premie!

Some information may seem new or surprising to you. However, every statement has firm scientific evidence behind it. A number inside brackets in the text, e.g. (2), refers to the "Fine Print Page" at the end of each chapter. This has comments by Dr Nils Bergman, and the scientific references. The fine print page is for you if you want more detail and it is also addressed to your doctor or nurse who can find the research-based evidence for what is being said.

I welcome your feedback and suggestions to make this book more helpful.

Jill Bergman
jill@kangaroomothercare.com
(November 2010)

Key pages are 10, 20, 26, 33, 44, 58, 77, 83 88, 94.

Hold Your Premie

a workbook on skin-to-skin contact
for parents of premature babies

by Jill Bergman, BA HDE

with

Dr Nils Bergman, MB ChB, DCH, MPH, MD
(USA equivalent MD, MPH, PhD)

To health professionals supporting parents with the help of this book

This book is primarily written to parents of preterm infants, but it is also written as a tool for you as health providers to support them.

There is a growing body of new evidence for best practices, some of which have turned our old beliefs upside down. There are many areas of controversy and others where evidence is insufficient or absent. However, parents want a distillation of the evidence, and how they can become part of best practice, just as much as we do as health professionals. In the process, some of the statements made in this book may seem over-simplified. My request is twofold: explain them better to your parents, and send your better explanation to us for future editions of this book.

It is not the intention that this book should cause conflict between health service providers on one hand, and parents making demands that cannot be met on the other. At the same time, this book does attempt to distill the latest available evidence from neuroscience and clinical studies, and in that way it does make demands on what best practice should look like. I am happy to be contacted concerning questions about references and quality of evidence, and how change processes can be facilitated. There is new evidence coming all the time and we should be continually prepared to adapt our care. The "Fine Print Pages" I have provided are a brief synopsis which I hope is helpful, and I am happy to develop these in future editions according to your suggestions.

Ideally we would see this book as a shared journey for parents and staff. Some parents may grasp the concepts without help, but the primary intention is that they should be able to work through the book with guidance and support from you as health professionals. For example, the chapters on "Technology" and "Problems Premies May Face" are purposefully brief, the tables are there to facilitate your interaction with the parents, each baby and each situation is unique. That way every parent, regardless of reading level, will get most benefit, and you will explain things relevant to your own hospital context.

The greatest challenge embodied in this book lies in the changing role of parents in the care of premature infants. In the past, they were excluded from the NICU completely, and our health systems and our infrastructure were designed accordingly. Allowing them back can be practically difficult; giving them centre stage can seem overwhelming. But on this point we should not compromise, future quality of care for prematurity will be measured in terms of emotional, social and neurodevelopmental outcomes. Improving these requires parental presence and involvement in care: mother is the key to optimal neurodevelopment.

Dr Nils Bergman
nils@kangaroomothercare.com
(November 2010)

CONTENTS

HOW TO USE THIS BOOK   iv

INTRODUCTION   7

THE FIRST FEW HOURS   10

HOW PREMIES ARE DIFFERENT FROM FULL-TERM NEWBORNS   20

WHAT PARENTS CAN DO TO HELP THEIR BABY   26

EMOTIONS AND COPING   33

SKIN-TO-SKIN CONTACT   44

BREASTMILK AND BREASTFEEDING   58

WAYS OF FEEDING PRETERM BABIES   65

BREASTFEEDING YOUR PRETERM BABY   72

HOW THE BRAIN DEVELOPS AND WORKS: NEUROSCIENCE   77

PROTECT SLEEP   83

SEPARATION AND STRESS   88

DEVELOPMENTAL CARE   94

TECHNOLOGY   108

PROBLEMS PREMIES MAY FACE IN THE NICU   121

LONG TERM PROBLEMS PREMIES MAY FACE & HOW
SKIN-TO-SKIN CONTACT CAN HELP   124

HOW FRIENDS AND FAMILY CAN HELP   129

GOING HOME   131

PARENTING   135

COMPASSIONATE CARE FOR A DYING BABY   142

RESOURCES   145

INTRODUCTION

Many parents come to me after a talk on prematurity and say

"If only I'd known…I would have done things differently."

Any mother or father who has sat watching their little premie in an incubator struggling to breathe knows that feeling of utter helplessness and despair, and the agony of leaving their tiny baby so alone in hospital. But there is an alternative which can turn this situation to hope! It is "skin-to-skin contact".

HOLD YOUR PREMIE

This book is for you parents who find yourselves in the scary, confusing situation of having a preterm baby. Some bigger and full term babies may go to the Neonatal Intensive Care Unit (NICU) if they are sick or need special care. All of the information given is valid for these babies and their parents too.

There are countless parenting books in the bookstores. There is as much advice out there as there are women and grannies in the world! But almost all of the advice given is from the parents' perspective! Yes, parents like to have their sleep and their "well-behaved baby" and will buy the books that promise them what they want. Unfortunately, this is very often not what the baby needs and wants.

This is a baby-centered book, based on the baby's basic biological needs, both physical and emotional. In particular, it speaks for the premature newborn, who cannot speak for herself.

This is a workbook and has been written to help you to help your baby. It gives simple information and practical things that you can do to be involved in the team that is caring for your premature baby.

There are so many different terms: premature baby, preterm infant, preemie, premie, etc; I will use the simplest, premie. Technically a "preterm" infant is anything less than 37 weeks completed gestational age, while a "premature" is one born before her organs are fully developed. As these terms are both used, I will use them interchangeably. I will also write as if the baby is a girl, as there are many cultures that do not value girls as highly as boys. Every baby is a gift!

Some of the statements in this book may seem challenging, but I have tried to describe practical ways to care for the newborn premie. The most recent research evidence all shows that the mother of the newborn is vitally important for her child's best development.

I also do not mean to make you as parents feel guilty if you were not able to do what you really wanted for your baby. I want you to have the evidence you need to empower you, and the tools to do all that you can to make up for your baby's rough start. No-one else and no artificial incubator can provide anything like mom's best care. The premie's own mother's milk provides food specific to the baby's needs. No artificial milk formula can ever come close!

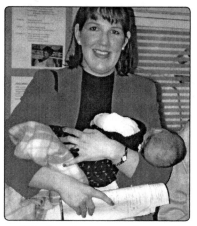

Personal testimony of a mother at International KMC Workshop

"The instinct of a mother to hold and care for her baby is primordial and primitive and an overwhelmingly powerful feeling."
Jane Davis, Bogota, Colombia, Dec 1998

It is natural to want to be with your baby.

It is right.

You, Mom, must trust your instinct of love and nurture.

The bond between the newborn child and mother is vital and forms the basis for all relationships later. Why has this changed so much lately? What will the impact of this be on the present and future generations?

The fierceness with which she protects her young is the measure of how good an animal mother is. It is her natural maternal instinct and it is needed for the survival of her baby.

It will be your natural instinct to protect your baby too. But often in our technological age you as parents may feel paralyzed and disempowered by the sight of all the machinery in a NICU. You may feel worry, fear, confusion and uncertainty. You may feel very vulnerable at this stage as you want the best for your baby and you may think that an incubator is what your baby needs. The machines are needed but you are needed even more!

As a new parent of a premie, you need to know that you are not alone, that there are many other new parents who are feeling the same worry and trauma as you are (about one in eight babies in the world is born prematurely). Each mother and father will have different feelings, each hospital and clinic situation will be different; each premature baby will have her own unique complications of being born too early.

The technology that we have in the modern world is amazing and wonderful, and your baby should have access to all the technology that she needs to survive. The younger she is, the more machinery is needed. While technology ensures survival, what we also need to understand is what modern neuroscience is discovering; for the best quality survival and for brain development the premie baby needs mother to be present.

This is written for all parents of all premies, whether in a high-tech NICU or places with less resources, because the babies' basic biological needs are the same. In places that do not have access to first world technology, giving skin-to-skin contact alone may save the baby's life (1). In a NICU where people have access to incubators and all of the machines needed, knowing this information will help them to give all of the technological support needed, but in the right place: on the mother's chest.

Interestingly many cases have been recorded of very small babies who were not expected to survive who were put on their mothers' chest. These babies started to dramatically improve and even grew faster than the incubator babies! This convinced hospitals to do skin-to-skin contact. Susan Ludington-Hoe starts her book with one such example (2).

In the past babies needed to be stable in incubators before parents were allowed to touch or hold their babies. However, there is no technical definition for what a "stable" baby is. Secondly, there is clinical evidence that shows that a baby becomes more stable more quickly on her mother's chest (3). You may need to find new ways and ask for your baby to get all the technical support she needs while she is on your chest.

> **<u>The aim is to keep mother and baby together as much as possible.</u>**
> **Mother is the key to the best development for the premature baby.**
> **The science behind this shows that:**
> 1. **the mother provides all the sensory stimulation needed for the brain of the baby to grow;**
> 2. **skin-to-skin contact is the best way to provide ideal care, it provides all the body's needs.**
> 3. **technology should be added as required; it is not a substitute for the mother.**

This book will help you understand the technology your baby needs and give you practical ways to help your premie's development so that later problems are reduced as far as possible.

If you are likely to have a preterm baby, try to read this before your baby is born to get those first hours right. This will make things easier for you and your baby. If your baby is already in a NICU, you may not have much time; read the first page of each chapter. Read the other sections as you need them.

It is my hope and prayer that this information will lessen the stress of having a premature baby and that it will help you and your premie to cope better.

THE FIRST FEW HOURS

- Skin-to-skin contact should start at birth, or as soon after that as possible.

- This is for <u>all</u> babies, and even more so for premies.

- This helps them stabilize their heart rate, breathing and temperature.

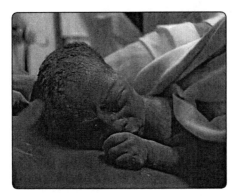

Mom, ask for your naked baby to be put on your naked chest straight after delivery in the labor ward (4).

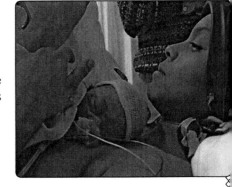

She can be dried off and both of you can be covered together. All the tests and assessments can be done while she is on your chest.

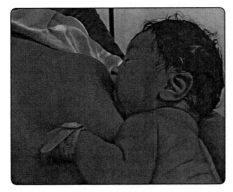

She should stay naked on your chest for at least the first hour; she should not be taken away or bathed during that time. It is very likely that your baby will smell and make her own way to your nipple and try to latch on (5). Encourage her. Your baby should not be suctioned at this time as it will disturb her suckling reflex (6).

As your baby is born, she needs you, her mother.

You provide the sensations which make your baby feel safe; this in turn encourages her stability.

The brain of the baby has been developing from very early in pregnancy. During the last third of the pregnancy, the brain development is huge. For all full term babies this usually happens inside the mother, and this is what the baby expects biologically. If your baby is born premature, this brain development will be occurring in the NICU which is NOT ideal, and we need to minimize the shock for her.

Skin-to-skin contact provides the biologically expected stimulation to wire the brain in the best way possible. At the same time, the skin-to-skin contact between mom and baby is the way that the mother's 'autonomic nervous system' (ANS) helps the baby's body to find balance.

The brain is stimulated by sensations. Sensations from the mother are good and reassuring. They make the brain develop. As time passes, new sensations stimulate new parts of the brain to connect. This brain-wiring depends on mother's presence. Look for more detail in the chapter on Neuroscience, see page 77.

AT BIRTH YOUR BABY NEEDS and expects to

1. feel your skin against hers, keeping her warm and you holding her tight;

2. smell you (this is one of her first senses to develop);

3. hear your voice and heartbeat (she's heard them for months – both will soothe her);

4. see you! (she knows what a face is and looks for you);

5. taste your breast and later your milk.

SENSATIONS THAT WIRE BRAIN

SEES Mom's eyes
Ear HEARS Mom's voice
SMELLS Mom's milk
MOVES with Mom
TASTES Mom's milk
Back FEELS Mom's arm holding
Hands TOUCH Mom's skin
Skin-to-skin CONTACT
WARMED on Mom's front

The technology that separates a mom and her premie deprives the baby's brain of the sensations needed for healthy brain development.

An "incubator" is what is used to hatch chickens! The incubator name "Isolette" shows that the baby is isolated from her mom and dad. This is not a good thing – she needs you, her parents.

Skin-to-skin contact with your baby

0–90 minutes after birth	is essential for her best brain development, physically and mentally.
0–6 hours after birth	will help her cardio-respiratory (heart and breathing) systems to physically stabilize.
6–24 hours after birth	helps the baby to get into a stable feeding pattern and sleep cycling.
12 hours to 8 weeks after birth	is essential for attachment and bonding.

Skin-to-skin contact can be started many days after birth if it has not been possible before. Many premies are born with problems and complications of various kinds which need technological support. The key message is: **start as early as possible**. This will help you and your little one to bond closely and to help breastfeeding. She needs you to hold her close for weeks for her brain to grow properly. If you can only start this late, just continue longer!

As your baby is born

Your baby has been born too early and she is called a preterm or premature baby (premie). She has had a rough start; her brain is not fully developed, her lungs may not be ready for breathing air, her sight and hearing are extra sensitive, and her skin is extra fragile.

As you look at her you may think that she is far too tiny and delicate to touch, and you may worry whether she will survive. She may need machines to help her breathing, tubes in her nose or mouth for feeding, and heel pricks for blood tests. Nothing "nice" has happened to your baby. The doctors and nurses will do all they can to help her fight for her life, but you need to know that she needs you, her Mom and Dad more than anything else in the world.

You may wish that it was different, but I want to encourage you by showing that there is so much that you can do in these first hours and days of her life that may even mean

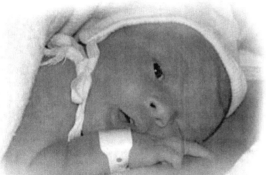

life or death for her. Most of all, it is the long-term **quality** of life which is at stake. Helping her to be close to you will give her good physical and mental health now and a better foundation for her development.

Your baby has been safe inside you for months, held close, warm and safe, hearing your heart beat and your voice. Your body has given her everything that she needs. Now that she is out in the big wide world too early, your job is to carry on giving her everything that she needs. Yes, you still can! She may need machines, but here are some practical things that you can do.

Practical:

It is very important to know that your tiny baby is YOUR tiny baby and she needs you. She longs to be held in skin-to-skin contact on your chest. **This is her safe place.** Ask the nurses to dry her gently and put her naked on your naked chest as she is born, and to cover both of you with a soft cloth and a blanket.

Your chest is the best place for your baby to adjust to life.

On your chest: **your baby will stay warmer and calmer,**
cry less, and
have better blood sugars
compared to being swaddled or put in a crib or an incubator (4).

> **Separation from you will cause your baby stress; gently and firmly insist that she stays with you.**

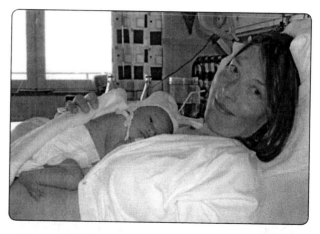

A premature baby cannot control her own body temperature properly and she may lose heat very quickly. Ask that she is not taken away and washed as this will make her temperature unstable; there is no benefit from bathing. The nurses and doctors can do many of their care procedures while she is safely and peacefully on your chest. Your hands are there to help hold her still. Hospitals have over the years developed technology and skills that rely on incubators. This requires adjusting and adapting to work on your chest, and sometimes the technology is such that this can't be done. When separation is needed, ask for your baby to be returned to you as soon as possible for you to settle her.

Ask that she is left on your chest for at least the first hour. Hold her as much as you can, for as long as you can. When she cries, the stress hormones in her body make her heart beat faster which sends more blood throughout her body. These stress hormones stay in the body for up to an hour. This uses up energy, and she needs all the energy she has to grow. If a tiny premie is stressed then her heart rate and blood pressure increases, this may cause the tiny blood vessels in the brain to burst (a brain bleed). Keep her calm in skin-to-skin contact to avoid this.

If your baby is extremely small, she may need CPAP, (continuous positive airways pressure) which is a way of providing extra pressure to each breath. If she is not managing on CPAP, she may need surfactant, or ventilation, and then the doctor may need to separate her from you. Your baby may also have medical conditions that need machinery that is not practical to do on your chest; the staff will explain this to you. You can then start working on a plan to get together again as soon as possible.

Skin-to-Skin Contact, cuddling and bonding help you and your baby to relate to each other better. Snuggling at birth gives you and your baby the best start for breast-feeding, and helps longer-term breastfeeding. These first few hours are important for "Self-Attachment". This is when newborn babies crawl without help up the mother's stomach to find and latch onto the breast. This happens best in the first hour after birth when the baby is awake and alert (5). If you have not had a chance to do this with your premie baby, be encouraged that it can happen even days after birth. Putting your baby in skin-to-skin contact on your chest and leaving her next to the breast will help breastfeeding to start normally. This is discussed in more detail in the chapter on breastfeeding. Attachment parenting is discussed in the chapter on the long-term benefits of skin-to-skin contact. Skin-to-skin babies are cuddled more even a year later.

Firm holding is what she needs next; after the first breastfeed. This is called "containment", and is very different to feather-light touch or stroking, which will irritate her sensitive skin. Inside your womb she was held very tightly, so bend her legs up close to her body with her arms close to her chest. Keep her hands near her mouth as she has been comforting herself like this for months. It helps "self-soothing" and will help her to be more peaceful and less stressed.

If you have had a caesarean section, dad or a nurse can support you to hold your premie on your chest. Alternatively, many hospitals will encourage dad to hold her skin-to-skin contact on his chest inside his shirt. She will know his voice from the months inside you and it is a wonderful time for dad to bond with his baby and to feel that he can help as well. (A dad will also feel helpless and worried when his baby is born too early, see page 26.) Remember that Skin-to-Skin Contact means no bra for mom and no clothes on your premie except a tiny nappy and your baby must be held under your shirt.

During skin-to-skin contact a wonderful thing can happen: your body temperature will automatically increase to warm your baby if she is cold and will cool down if your baby is hot! Your body's biology is wonderful! Studies have shown that for twins, a mom's breasts can have different temperatures depending on what each twin needs (7). Your body will keep your baby's temperature more stable than an incubator can. (This automatic temperature change does not work as well for dads (8). There is more for dads in a later chapter, see page 26.)

It is important that your premie does not become cold, for many reasons. One is that she has a chemical called "surfactant" in her lungs which help her to breathe. If she gets cold, this surfactant will not work so well and she will struggle to breathe. (She may also need to be given this surfactant to help her lungs work properly.) All first aid courses speak of A, B and C: airway, breathing and circulation. Your baby will need the same checkup as she is born. Your baby's tiny neck is not strong and her airway will need to be supported in the sniffing position to help her to breathe. As she has her first sleep she may need to be fixed onto your chest to stabilize her airway. She may need extra oxygen and she can get this through a tube while she is on your chest.

Your baby may need to be separated from you!

There are many reasons for premature birth and your baby may need to be taken to the NICU. Medical staff have traditionally stabilized babies in the incubator and the equipment is designed around it.

While in the incubator, your baby will probably not tolerate stroking and light touching very well. However the staff can show you how to hold your baby. Keep your hands still as you hold her feet against her body, or cup her head in your hand (for more see page 99).

Talk to your baby

Ask to sit in a chair next to your baby so you can hold her and talk to her. You can still hold her skin-to-skin when she has oxygen and heart monitors – this will help her to stabilize. It will also help you to feel like her mom and dad and to love her. (Parents of premies have not had all the usual months to prepare mentally for being parents, and need time to realize that they are parents to their very tiny baby.)

Once the difficult work is done on your baby, and the technology allows it, the baby can be moved back to your chest. The baby's condition will almost always benefit from this, but it is usually the technology as such which may prevent this from being possible. All technical support can be added when your premie is in skin-to-skin contact. This may mean systems changes in your NICU – encourage the nurses and doctors to look at the references on the "fine print pages" (9;10). This must also be done with the usual monitoring of "vital signs", which will confirm that the baby is recovering her balance (or stabilizing).

Your baby needs your breastmilk to give her the antibodies she needs to protect her. If you can, call in a lactation consultant or breastfeeding specialist to get your breastmilk started. If you do want to breastfeed, start pumping as soon as possible. You will have more success if you start within 6 hours of birth. Keeping your baby in skin-to-skin contact with her nuzzling your chest will help you to produce prolactin, the hormone which makes the milk.

If your baby is preterm, your milk will not be the same as the milk for a full term baby. Your body knows that it needs to produce breastmilk that will give your premie extra proteins for brain growth that she would have been getting through the umbilical cord. If she is a very tiny premie she may not yet be strong enough to suckle from your breast, but she still needs breastmilk. Express it and feed it to her through a tube in her nose or mouth that goes straight into her stomach. Feed her little amounts often as her stomach is so tiny. Express your milk more often and more milk will be produced. Even if there are only two drops of the early milk, colostrum, it will be enough to help her stomach to be healthy. Colostrum is called "liquid gold" because of all the antibodies that it contains to protect the tiny baby from germs. She does not need formula. Formula is milk designed for a baby cow and only has about 30 nutrients; your breastmilk will give her the thousands (literally!) of nutrients that a human baby needs for protection and for her brain to grow properly.

Sucking from a bottle is stressful and tiring for babies as they cannot breathe and suck from a bottle at the same time (11;12). Write on her card that she is not to be given a bottle. Feeding her your expressed milk in a tiny cup is better for her. Remember that your aim is to get her breastfeeding as soon as possible.

Premature babies need breast milk even more than full term babies to help them to grow properly and for their brains to grow healthy. With support, premies can breastfeed at 28 weeks.

Previously it was believed that premies could not breastfeed until 32 weeks gestation or a specific weight. Ask for a lactation consultant to help you get your baby to latch. Pay for her help if you need to; it is well worth getting help to start breastfeeding as your baby will have far fewer illness and allergy problems later in her life.

Your premie has been born too early and the first few hours may have been spent desperately trying to keep your tiny baby alive. Now she is breathing and her heart is working and feeding breast milk has started. You and your baby should continue to be one unit as you have been for months.

What do you do now?

It is time to evaluate the situation and find out what YOU as parents need.

Do you need more information on how to cope emotionally? You will find a chapter on this on page 33.

Maybe you want to find out more about the technology or medicines that your baby needs. Knowing more can make you feel less helpless. Ask the staff to explain what the wires and tubes connected to your baby are for. You can also start learning about the details of the technical support that premies may need (see page 108, the technology chapter). It is worth finding out as much as you can about your baby's needs and the medicines and machines that are helping her. You will be part of the team, and not just a victim or bystander.

Have you given your baby a name? Often, parents are too scared to do this in case their baby does not survive. Your baby has been a person for months already inside you. Give her a name: a name that you say softly to her whenever you spend time with her; her name that you say gently to comfort her. (You need to call her something as you speak to her ... perhaps you had a nickname for her while she was inside you ... maybe she even recognizes that for the time being!) Obviously this will depend on your cultural and religious traditions.

Have you shared your baby's arrival with your friends and family? They are more likely to be supportive if they know your news.

FIRST DAY CHECKLIST:

Have you given your child a name? ....

Have you taken her picture? ....

(Remember not to use a flash when taking photographs as this will hurt your premie's fragile eyes.)

Your own baby's FACT SHEET

Mom's name ....

Dad's name ....

Baby's name ....

Birth date ....

Time of birth ....

Weight at birth ....

Length at birth ....

Place of birth ....

Ask for your baby's diagnosis and medication to be written down for you

....

....

....

Baby's questions

How did you choose my name?

....

....

....

When did you first hold me? ....

When was my first breastfeed? ....

Doctors and nurses who helped me: ....

....

....

....

Use space below for handprint and footprint!

Parents' questions about NICU

Does your hospital allow skin-to-skin contact at birth?...

Does your NICU encourage skin-to-skin contact – or insist on it?...

For full term babies?.................................... For premies?..

Is there a place for you, her mom or dad to sit with your baby in skin-to-skin contact?

Can yiu sleep in the hospital if you have a premie baby?　　...

Fine Print Page - Introduction

This chapter summarizes many things, and the fine print on them will be found in later chapters. For example, the statements about your baby's brain needs, and separation, will be discussed in the fine print page in the Neuroscience chapter. Just for starters, here are some annotations.

1.   Without ventilators or incubators, but using mothers as incubators, survival improved from 10% to 50% in a study in Zimbabwe. Both authors were involved in developing the technique.

2.   This "dying infant" went on to survive. Care should be taken not to instil false hope for such "miracles" – See Compassionate Care chapter. However, if the baby improves, it deserves full care.

3.   In this randomized controlled trial, babies were between 1200g and 2200g. Those placed SSC from birth ALL stabilized after 6 hours, but only HALF those in incubators did so. The key is no separation, and starting from birth.

4.   The research on self-attachment started in Sweden, where researchers were studying how much warmth and extra sugar newborn babies needed. They found that undrugged babies that were left on their mom's chest all crawled by themselves unaided to the breast and started breastfeeding. After one hour, they had higher blood sugars than those given glucose, and they were much warmer.

5.   Dr Righard has produced a video of this work, available from www.geddesproduction.com   Dr Smillie has produced a video showing that this works days and weeks later, available same website.

6.   Suctioning "seemed unpleasant" and caused retching, and delayed breastfeeding behaviour.

7.   Susan Ludington has researched temperature effects on twins: "thermal synchrony" between mother and child ensures a very stable temperature, one degree higher than incubator.

8.   Dads tend to increase baby's temperature, but not dangerously, as the baby self-regulates by wriggling to cooler spots or putting out an arm.

9-10.   Here are detailed descriptions of techniques combining SSC and ventilation. Two of the most thorough covering many technical details are by Susan Ludington.

11-12.   There is a general belief that bottle is less stressful than breast, but there is no evidence to support this. Paula Meier researched this in 32 week infants who were bottle and breastfeeding; babies had lower oxygen both during and after bottle-feeding. Mizuno studied the musculature and pressures during both, and politely notes them to be different !

Reference List

(1)   Bergman NJ, Jurisoo LA. The 'kangaroo-method' for treating low birth weight babies in a developing country. Trop Doct 1994 April;24(2):57-60.

(2)   Ludington-Hoe SM. Kangaroo Care The best you can do for your infant. Bantam Books; 1993.

(3)   Bergman NJ, Linley LL, Fawcus SR. Randomized controlled trial of skin-to-skin contact from birth versus conventional incubator for physiological stabilization in 1200- to 2199-gram newborns. Acta Paediatr 2004 June;93(6):779-85.

(4)   Christensson K, Siles C, Moreno L, Belaustequi A, de la FP, Lagercrantz H et al. Temperature, metabolic adaptation and crying in healthy full-term newborns cared for skin-to-skin or in a cot. Acta Paediatrica (Oslo, Norway: 1992) 1992 June;81(6-7):488-93.

(5)   Righard L, Alade MO. Effect of delivery room routines on success of first breastfeed. Lancet 1990 November 3;336(8723):1105-7.

(6)   Widstrom AM, Ransjo-Arvidson AB, Christensson K, Matthiesen AS, Winberg J, Uvnas-Moberg K. Gastric suction in healthy newborn infants. Effects on circulation and developing feeding behaviour. Acta Paediatr Scand 1987 July;76(4):566-72.

(7)   Ludington-Hoe Sm, Lewis T, Morgan K, Cong X, Anderson L, Reese S. Breast-infant temperature synchrony with twins during shared kangaroo care. JOGNN 2006;35(2):1-9.

(8)   Ludington-Hoe SM, Hashemi MS, Argote LA, Medellin G, Rey H. Selected physiologic measures and behavior during paternal skin contact with Colombian preterm infants. J Dev Physiol 1992 November;18(5):223-32.

(9)   Ludington-Hoe Sm, Ferreira C, Swinth J, Ceccardi JJ. afe Criteria and Procedure for Kangaroo Care with intubated Preterm Infants. JOGNN 2007;32(2003):579-88.

(10)   Ludington-Hoe Sm, Morgan K, Abouelfettah A. A clinical guideline for implemetation of kangaroo care with premature infants of 30 or more weeks' postmenstrual age. Advances in Neonatal Care 2008;8(3 S):S3-S23.

(11)   Meier P. Bottle- and breastfeeding: effects on transcutaneous oxygen pressure and temperature in preterm infants. Nursing Research 1988 January;37(1):36-41.

(12)   Mizuno K, Ueda A. Changes in Sucking Performance from Nonnutritive Sucking to Nutritive Sucking during Breast-and-Bottle-Feeding. Pediatr Res 2006;59(5):728-7.

HOW PREMIES ARE DIFFERENT FROM FULL-TERM NEWBORNS

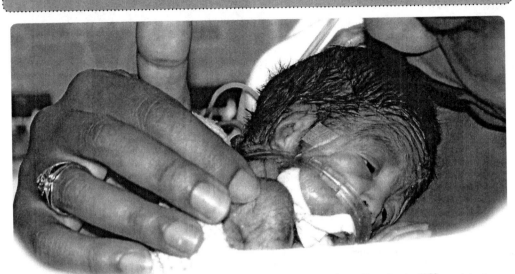

You may get a shock when you first see your baby: premies often look different to term babies. She has not had time to grow in size and put on weight and be nicely rounded.

Be reassured; she will grow to look "normal" in time.

She may look:

- very tiny, like a little wizened old woman with a wrinkled face.
- Her head may look too large for her body size and be longer and thinner. Her head bones are soft.
- Her body and head are big but her skinny arms may make her look like an underfed child.
- Her ribs may stick out, and may cave in with each breath.
- Her arms and legs often look too long and too thin and will often be straight out, not bent or flexed.
- Her skin is thin, fragile and shiny, and wrinkled. Her skin may change color depending on the amount of oxygen in her blood.
- Your premie's eyes may stay closed because her eyes are so sensitive to light.
- Your premie's hands and feet are often perfectly formed, just long and thin.
- Her ears may be very soft and unformed.
- She may have hair on her body, especially the shoulders.
- She may need lots of tubes and machines to help her survive as her tiny body may not be ready to cope on her own. This is often the most scary thing for parents to see.

Inside the premature baby the body systems are immature.

- Her heart may beat very irregularly.
- Her lungs may struggle to breathe.
- Her central nervous system is immature so she may twitch more.
- Her digestive system may take time to work properly.
- Your premie's immune system is immature and will need your colostrum or first milk to help protect her.

A full-term baby would have 40 weeks inside the mother where all her needs are provided. As a full-term baby is born, huge changes are needed for the new-born to cope in her new environment. For a premie, these adjustments for heart, lungs, temperature and immune and metabolic control can be overwhelming, or life-threatening.

Changes to life outside the womb are more difficult for your premie to make.

Premies are "pre-mature" babies. They are born too early and are not fully ready to make the adjustments to life outside the mother. The premie of 24 weeks gestation should have had another 16 weeks in her mother's womb. With improved technology and feeding, preterm babies are surviving at earlier and earlier ages. In the past, neonatal care was focused on survival. This meant support was needed for the immature body and her developing lungs and heart. Modern neonatal care (and this book!) is now focusing on the quality of survival, and how to improve the long term brain development to achieve a good future for each child.

There are two main measures of fetal development, namely age and weight. Full gestation is regarded as 40 weeks (nine months plus one week). Any early birth from 24 weeks to 37 weeks gestation is a preterm birth. Technically, babies 37 weeks and above are not seen as being preterm. Generally, the longer the tiny developing baby stays in her mother's womb, the better she can cope – inside mom is where her body is designed to grow best. Generally, the more premature the baby is, the more problems she has. The gestational age is usually assessed before birth, but can also be measured by scoring certain physical features. Weight is less important, but generally the lower the weight, the more problems the premie faces. Babies can be both premature and small for their age (see page 25).

Abbreviations:	Translated	Meaning
GA	Gestational Age	The weeks from conception to birth
SGA	Small for Gestational Age	A premature baby who is too small for her gestational age (because of malnutrition, mother smoking, etc.)
AGA	Appropriate for Gestational Age	A premie baby is smaller than a full term, but the right size for her gestational age
LBW	Low birth weight.	baby below 5.5 lbs (2,5kg)
VLBW	Very low birth weight	below 3.3lbs (1500g)
ELBW	Extremely low birth weight	below 2.2lbs (1000g)

What your baby looks like will depend on how many weeks premature she was born.

She has been born early and is <u>very</u> tiny. If she is more than 8 weeks premature she may look very different to a full term baby and may need high-tech assistance to help breathing.

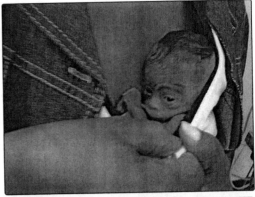

As you look at her it may be a shock as she has not had time to grow in size and put on weight and be nicely rounded. Some parents say their premies look like little wizened old women. It may be a shock to see how tiny she is, but look at her perfect fingers and toes – she is "fearfully and wonderfully made".

Some parents of premies comment on the wonder of being able to watch their baby grow; if she had not been born early they would not have been able to see that development.

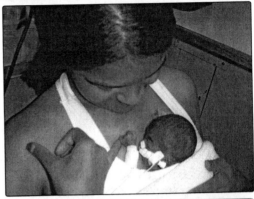

<u>The premie's head</u> often looks larger than normal in relation to her body size. She loses most of her heat through her head so she may need to wear a cap all the time.

If a premie is in an incubator, her head may not stay rounded instead become longer and thinner, Her head can also become flattened as the skull bones are still soft.

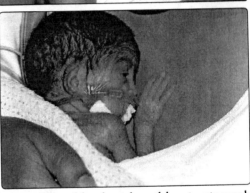

<u>Body</u>: her body is big and her head is big but her skinny arms may make her look like an underfed child. Her ribs often stick out and may cave in with each breath. This chest breathing is a sign of stress. She may struggle to breathe as her lungs are immature and she may need help from a ventilator. As she grows she will change from this chest breathing to stomach breathing which is better. Even tiny premies change to this stable abdominal breathing when they have Skin-to-Skin Contact.

<u>Arms and legs</u>: the arms and legs often look too long and too thin as the fat tissue has not been put in place. The arms and legs will often be straight out, not flexed.

<u>Skin</u>: her skin is thin, fragile and shiny. The color depends on what is happening underneath the skin. If she has good oxygenation, then the premie is rosy and pink. Premies often look blue as they struggle to get enough oxygen. Premies don't have a layer of stored fat under their skin so the skin often looks wrinkled. It may also look wrinkled if the baby has lost fat. SGA babies may have needed to use some of their stored fat before they were born if the placenta was not working properly (for example). ELBW babies have skin that leaks water. These "aquapores" close after 1–2 days.

Hair on the body: between 28 weeks and 36 weeks of development, the human baby often has hair called lanugo on the shoulders and back. This is normal and will disappear in time.

Eyes: a premie's eyes may stay closed because they are so sensitive to light (especially if she is below 30 weeks). Between 30–34 weeks the pupil will begin to constrict to limit the amount of light coming into the eye. If you close curtains, dim the lights and hold your baby skin-to-skin, she will often open her eyes.

Hands and feet: the premie's hands and feet are often perfectly formed, just long and thin. If the baby is born before 24 weeks there are often no creases on the soles of the feet, or on the hands. Often the premie's toenails and fingernails are not yet formed. These signs help doctors to score the baby's age.

Ears: only from 28 weeks onwards does the outer ear begin to stiffen as the cartilage of the ear does not develop before then. Before 35 weeks your premie's ears may be floppy. Ear development also helps doctors score the age of the baby.

Muscles: premie babies often have low muscle tone and so appear "floppy".

Genitalia: these may be very underdeveloped in a premie and may look strange. Do not worry; they will develop normally in time.

The premature baby has immature body systems.

There are many reasons for prematurity. Your premie's need for specific support and technology will depend on her gestational age and stability. Each premie's needs are unique. You as parents need to know about the various organs and systems.

- Heart
- Lungs
- Central Nervous system
- Endocrine system
- Digestive system
- Immune system

The body is still preparing for birth so the lungs, gut and kidneys need to continue to develop.

A baby's lungs expect to mature just before birth at 40 weeks. It is the stress of being born that helps them to mature As she has been born early, the premie's lungs are not fully developed and she may need help from machines for breathing, extra oxygen or surfactant. Steroids are often given to mothers at risk for preterm birth, to help the baby's lungs to mature faster.

You need to understand the technology that is helping your baby to survive. I will translate the technical words used in the NICU in a later chapter.

Inside her mother the fetus has:

- oxygen and food that are provided through the placenta;
- no need to breathe or digest;
- a stable temperature;
- a safe place to curl up;

constant gentle sounds – mom's heartbeat, muffled voices and other sounds;

the day – night rhythms of her mom;

no need to respond to lots of messages and distractions – her nervous system is protected;

no lights.

<u>Outside mother the premie</u> is not able to regulate her own body, and so:

<u>Physically:</u>

her heart rate and breathing are uneven;

she changes color often.

she is tense, her muscles twitch and she trembles;

she is likely to be stiff, but she may be limp;

she can't stay curled up.

she gets tired quickly;

<u>Emotionally:</u>

she can't be alert;

she is fussy and unsettled;

she can't focus on you for a long time;

she struggles to calm down after being disturbed.

<u>What a difference Skin-to-Skin Contact can make!</u>

Mom and Dad, you can help your baby's body temperature to stay constant, and her breathing and heart rate to stabilize. You are absolutely essential for your premie's best care, so make the time now to be there for your baby. Both parents are needed so that there is less stress caused by separation.

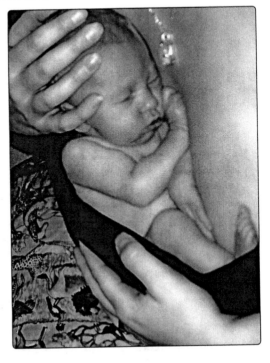

You can use this diagram to better understand your premie's development.
Using baby's weight and age, follow the instruction in the middle of the diagram.

Your baby's birth weight ....

Her gestational age ....

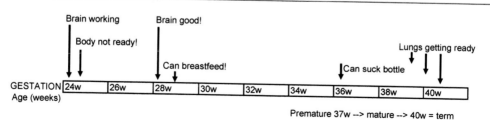

Brain working   Brain good!

Body not ready!

Can breastfeed!   Lungs getting ready

                                    Can suck bottle

GESTATION Age (weeks)	24w	26w	28w	30w	32w	34w	36w	38w	40w

Premature 37w --> mature --> 40w = term

ELBW ———➤   VLBW ———➤   LBW ———➤

WEIGHT at birth		1000g 2.2 lb		1500g 3.3 lb		2500g 5.5 lb		

Temp control:
begins --> okay
1800g --> 2200g

Mark an "X" on the gestation age scale for your own baby
Then mark an "X" for the birth weight of your own baby.
Now draw an arrow from the top "X" to the bottom "X"

GESTATION Age (weeks)	24w	26w	28w	30w	32w	34w	36w	38w	40w

WEIGHT at birth	800g 1lb 12oz	900g 2lb	1100g 2lb 7oz	1300g 2lb 14oz	1700g 3lb 12oz	2000g 4lb 6 oz	2600g 5lb 12oz	2900g 6lb 6oz	3200g 7lb 1oz

If the arrow points straight down, then your baby is normal, or usual, weight for that womb age.
If the arrow leans a little bit in either direction, it is also probably normal.
If the arrow leans more backwards, (down to the left), then your baby is small for its gestation
If the arrow leans forward (down to the right), then your baby is large for its gestation.

WHAT PARENTS CAN DO TO HELP THEIR BABY

Mom and Dad, you can both do so much for your baby.

The most important things are to:

- ☐ BE THERE WITH HER
- ☐ HOLD YOUR PREMIE
- ☐ GET INVOLVED IN HER CARE

Mom's chest provides the place for the smoothest transition from life in the womb to life in the world. It is the safe place where all of your baby's needs can be met. Mom provides emotional continuity of love, security and relationship so that her baby does not become stressed.

A baby is more stable on her mother's chest than in an incubator. The more premature the baby is, the more she needs her mother to reach stability.

Even a 28 week premie can breathe properly on her mother's chest, can breastfeed properly, and all her body systems can adapt better to her new life.

Skin-to-Skin Contact and breastfeeding provide stability for the newborn. The mother's body provides the continuity of sensations that the baby's brain needs, and the baby's brain in turn controls the body of the baby.

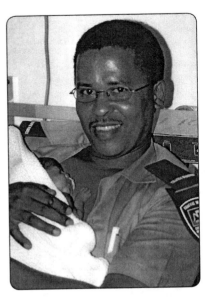

<u>Dads have a vital role to play:</u>

You can hold your baby skin-to-skin, especially if Mom has had a Caesarean section.

You can feed her through a tube or cup-feed her the breastmilk.

You can change diapers, bathe her, etc.

The only thing dad can't do is breastfeed!

ON PARENT'S CHEST: 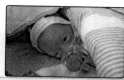	INCUBATOR: (SEPARATED) 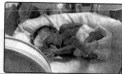
Unstressed baby	Stressed baby
Respiratory Rate more even	Breathing often irregular
Heart rate normal & stable	Heart Rate very variable or slower
Temperature slightly higher than incubator and in a very small range	Big fluctuations in temperature
Self attachment and bonding	Protest and crying
Breastfeeding and growth	Dissociation and survival and less growth
Breastmilk provides immune protection and nutritional needs	No immune protection at all from cow's milk, and only basic nutritional needs are provided
Best sensory stimulation so the baby has emotional well-being	Harmful stimuli to the brain
Absorbs food in the gut well	Gut absorption has shut down
Grows faster (> 2/3 oz/day)	Grows slower (1/3 oz/day)

Dad: you have a vital role to play in the life of your premature infant!

This section is addressed to fathers, but I know that in some situations fathers may be absent or not be part of this process. This may bring up its own set of issues and emotions to deal with. Get help if you need it. The broader family and friends can be a wonderful support.

How a dad can help his baby:

Nothing can properly prepare you for the time of watching your tiny baby struggling to breathe or lying on her back with tubes and lines and monitors all over her tiny body. But if you hold her on your chest you experience being her father! You can do so much for her! Your baby will recognize your voice from all those months inside mom. Talk to her if she is in an incubator, and you can also carry her skin-to-skin. If possible, hold your baby while mom recovers from a caesarean section. This can be a wonderful and beautiful time as you bond with your tiny baby. Your baby needs you – and so does the mother of your baby.

You may be shocked at her premature birth and feel absolutely helpless. It is normal and OK to feel like this. It is normal to go through a whole range of scary emotions. I will explain these later in the workbook (see page 33). What is very important is that you allow yourself to feel these emotions and express them. Do not try to deny what you are feeling. It can be very frustrating not being in control of the situation, especially if you feel that you have to take responsibility for your family. You may feel angry or

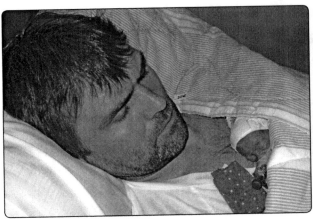 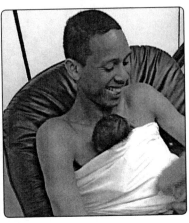

helpless. You need to be involved, find out as much as possible about your premie and her medications. Ask for professional help if you are not coping.

You can share in providing all your baby's care. There are only two things you cannot do. First, you can't breastfeed! However your baby may suck on your nipple, though this might be embarrassing, it is okay. If mom is nearby, move baby to her breast. Secondly, your temperature may not adjust as the mother's does when you hold your premie in Skin-to-Skin Contact (1). Dads tend to overheat their babies, but that is usually not a problem as your baby will stick out an arm to cool herself down. If you are holding your baby, do not put a cap on her. Otherwise, you can do everything just as well as mom (2;3).

You can:

- Feed your baby expressed breastmilk through a nasogastric tube, syringe, or cup
- Hold your baby in skin-to-skin contact as she sleeps
- Help with nesting and positioning to make her comfortable if she has to be in an incubator
- Find information on websites about medications and machines your baby needs
- Read baby's medical charts and ask staff to explain your baby's condition
- Be supportive to mom
- Encourage staff to give your baby developmental care
- Be the Protector and Champion for your baby to get the very best care possible for her!

Helping baby's mom:

You can help your partner by reading this book and discussing each chapter!

When you get involved, mom will be relieved and feel that you are lifting her load.

Share your feelings with your wife or partner and share the experience. It is a difficult time for any relationship and you will need to keep communicating. It can be hard to be apart if mom stays in hospital but try to find times when you can be together. Your wife or partner

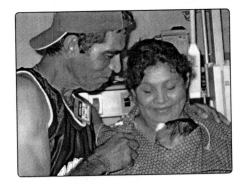

may be emotionally upside-down because of hormones or extreme stress. BE there for her and share it with her. One important thing that you can do is to reassure her. She may feel that your baby being born too early is her "fault". It is not. Support her and do not blame her.

Dad, if you have other small children at home just being at home with them may be the most wonderful support you can give.

Sometimes you can hold your premie baby in Skin-to-Skin Contact while her mother goes home to rest or to give attention to another child.

In many parts of the world, dads are doing a lot of the Skin-to-Skin Contact. In Sweden, where there is a strong social security system and dads are given a lot of paternity leave, dads and moms often share the 24 hours of Skin-to-Skin Contact between them. It is also almost routine

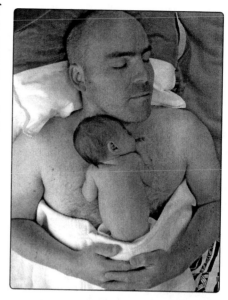

for dad to hold his baby after caesarean section (4). These dads have reported that the time each spent with their premie in Skin-to-Skin Contact in the NICU has formed a very special bond with his baby which will be the basis of a trusting relationship all her life.

Find ways of helping with the simple, practical care of your baby, including giving feeds before baby is able to breastfeed (5). Often, a dad is able to react more practically and technically in the time soon after a premie birth, as this is developing a new relationship with your child, (Mom is still feeling the loss of her pregnancy) (6;7).

Based on the reading above, what would be your next step to help your premie?

....

....

....

And after that, what will you do?

....

....

....

....

....

....

Benefits of Skin-to-Skin Contact for dads!

— You are empowered to care for your baby and do not feel helpless or useless,

— You are central to the caring team,

— Better bonding,

— Emotional healing,

— You are calmer and more relaxed,

— You are able to read your baby's unique cues for hunger or stress,

— You can get more sleep.

This section has covered the unexpected premature birth, and the next chapter looks at the rollercoaster of emotions that you may go through. Your baby is dependent on you to be involved early on, and to work through these issues with the support of your family.

Write down some of your own thoughts or experiences in the space below if you wish. You may never have done this kind of thing before. Try it! If you are used to doing this, continue to journal. You may not remember this time in NICU in future, but may find this record valuable. Maybe you will even share it with your child when she is older!

....

....

....

....

....

....

....

....

....

....

....

....

....

....

Are you artistic? What about making a sketch of your baby?

Take photos of her but remember not to use the flash as the bright light will hurt her sensitive eyes.

Fine Print Page

This page is only about fathers, the evidence in the summary on mothers will come in other chapters. There is surprisingly little research done on dads during the period before and after birth, and even less on fathers doing Skin-to-Skin Contact.

1. Susan Ludington has been mentioned already, in her study fathers warmed their babies too well!
2. German researchers have studied babies between 28 and 31 weeks, just 11 babies, but measured in detail. They concluded there was no real difference on mom or dad in oxygen consumption, carbon dioxide produc-tion, energy expenditure, skin and rectal temperatures, heart and respiratory rates, arterial saturation, and be-havioral states. They found "no adverse effects", and from reports both parents provide long periods of SSC to their pre-mies in most German NICU's.
3. The Swedish researchers mentioned earlier studied babies after caesarean section managed in cot compared to father's skin. They reported that the blood glucose levels while on fathers skin in the first 2 hours actually in-creased ... and it could not have been due to breastfeeding!! The temperatures were also higher than when cared for in a cot or an incubator, and surprisingly they were higher even 24 hours later.
4. This paper describes greatly reduced infant crying while on father's skin, with infants falling asleep after one hour.
5. Being involved practically, in this paper with feeding specifically, was an important element in paternal-infant bonding.
6. Mothers and fathers were interviewed about their reactions to premature birth. Both were taken by surprise, but fathers were more "ready to be involved immediately". For mothers the premie birth meant a "temporar-ily lost relationship", but for fathers this was new relationship just starting.
7. A hand book for fathers – not just for dads of preterms.

Reference List

(1) Ludington-Hoe SM, Hashemi MS, Argote LA, Medellin G, Rey H. Selected physiologic measures and behav-ior during paternal skin contact with Colombian preterm infants. J Dev Physiol 1992 November;18(5):223-32.

(2) Bauer J, Sontheimer D, Fischer C, Linderkamp O. Metabolic rate and energy balance in very low birth weight infants during kangaroo holding by their mothers and fathers. J Pediatr 1996 October;129(4):608-11.

(3) Christensson K. Fathers can effectively achieve heat conservation in healthy newborn infants. Acta Paediatr 1996 November;85(11):1354-60.

(4) Erlandsson K, Dsilna A, Fagerberg I, Christensson K. Skin-to-Skin Care with the Father after Cesarean Birth and Its Effect on Newborn Crying and Prefeeding Behavior. Birth: Issues in Perinatal Care 2007 June;34(2):105-14.

(5) Taubenheim AM. Paternal--infant bonding in the first-time father. JOGN Nursing; Journal Of Obstetric, Gyneco-logic, And Neonatal Nursing 1981 July;10(4):261-4.

(6) Fegran L, Helseth S, Fagermoen MS. A comparison of mothers' and fathers' experiences of the attachment proc-ess in a neonatal intensive care unit. Journal of Clinical Nursing 2008 March 15;17(6):810-6.

(7) Houser PM. Fathers-To-Be Handbook: A road map for the transition to fatherhood. 1st ed. South Portland, Maine 04106: Creative Life Systems; 2009.

EMOTIONS AND COPING

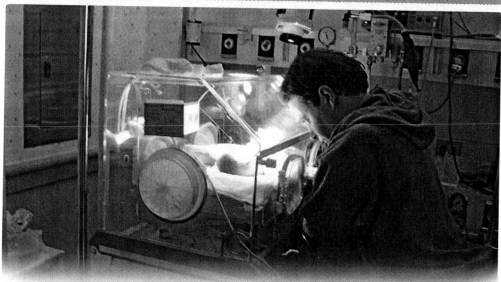

Nothing can fully prepare you for parenting a premie.

You have to learn on the job.

There are many things you can do, but the key things are
- Get involved in caring for your baby.
- Talk to other parents, talk to counselors, a social worker or a nurse
- CRY
- Ask for support and help if it feels like too much.

You may be overwhelmed by having a premie baby. It may be very scary for you worrying if your baby will survive. It is normal and OK to have these upside-down feelings and emotions. As parents you may both be under huge strain and worry. Try to keep sharing your feelings and supporting each other. It is also important to face the feelings and work through them so that you can help your baby.

Ask for help if you are struggling.

Your child needs a name!!

Some parents do not want to name their child, because they do not want to bond with her in case she dies. But your baby desperately needs you to bond with her and needs your love, your prayers, your longing for her, to help her to survive.

Many parents of premies have not had the last few weeks of pregnancy to finalize the choice of a name but it is very important.

Mothers and fathers usually have 9 months of pregnancy to prepare themselves mentally and emotionally for their new baby. When their baby is born early they are not ready or prepared. If it has been a high risk pregnancy or they are expoecting twins, parents may have had some time to prepare, but that is also very stressful. There may have been problems with mom's health and she may already have spent days or weeks in hospital.

At the onset of preterm labor, there is often a lot of anxiety and fear. Many parents describe their dream of having the suitcases packed and the baby's room decorated ready to receive her being shattered as they drive to the hospital. Something is wrong and your baby is being born prematurely. As this is often a time when doctors and nurses are desperately working to keep your baby alive, they may not have time to give you all the information you need. The first view of your tiny baby may be very scary (see page 20). She looks so very small and frail, and not at all like the full-term baby that you were expecting. She may be wrinkled, have hair on her shoulders, tubes in her nose and be attached to all sorts of machines that you haven't yet learnt about. She may be struggling to breathe, and be silent, or have a very weak cry. This image of her burns its way into your mind. Somehow you need to face the reality that this tiny premie baby is your child. It is normal to wish that it was different, but try to bring your mind back to the present. You need to accept the situation <u>as it is and do all you can</u> to make the best of it.

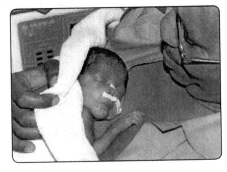

<u>Have you given your child a name?</u>
This is very important in terms of coping emotionally.

It is also very scary when you wonder if your child will survive. Some parents do not want to name their child, because they do not want to bond with her in case she dies. This is inside-out thinking – your baby desperately needs you to bond with her. She needs your love, your prayers, your longing for her to help her to survive. She needs to know she is wanted, to help her frail and tiny body to fight for life.

Your baby has been born too early and is too small – it is a confusing, frightening time and there is always the big question –

Will my baby survive?

This manual is intended to help you navigate through the scary and confusing weeks while your child is in the NICU and to help you so that you can help your baby.

Every family is unique, each premie has her own, sometimes complex problems, and is slightly different from other premies, your uncertainty of the future can be increased by not understanding the medical jargon. There may also be a lot of stress around the time of discharge from the hospital – "will I cope on my own?" In the case of bereavement, if your baby dies, it is even harder to bear. (This is covered at the back of this book, see page 142.)

Your emotions will swing and be unstable; partly because your hormones are changing, but also because this is a major life shock. You will probably go through some or all of the following emotions, not necessarily in this order, and some many times over (1)!

At this time, you may feel:

- Overwhelming shock
- Disbelief or denial
- Grief
- Anticipatory grief
- Fear
- Guilt
- A sense of failure
- Anger
- Confusion
- Depressed and cry a lot
- Immense strain
- Upset with nurses

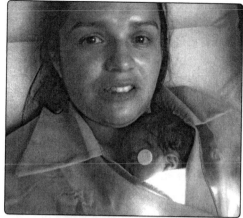

You may also find it

- Difficult to concentrate
- Difficult to sleep

<u>Here are some of the details</u>

You may feel overwhelming shock at the early birth.

<u>Disbelief or denial</u> is often a defense mechanism to stop you from attaching to an infant that may not survive.

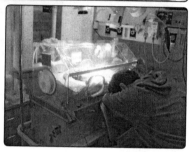

<u>Grief</u> is not just grief when someone dies; in the case of a premie baby the mother and father may go through what is called "anticipatory grief", which is looking at the possibility of death of their tiny baby. As parents you may fear that she won't survive, so you may be reluctant to bond with her. Yet she desperately needs you to bond with her and love her to help her gain strength for survival. Parents may also grieve the loss of a successful pregnancy, and the loss of a dream or expectation of a healthy full-term baby. (2)

Linked to this, mom (specifically) may feel <u>guilty</u>, or feel that she is a failure. She may <u>blame</u> herself for having done something wrong, or not being "a good enough mother" to deliver a "normal" baby. Most of this feeling is false guilt. Some moms – after reading this – may feel guilty that they did not care for their premies in the best way. It is never too late to give your baby extra love! <u>Self-doubt</u> drains a lot of energy and is not helpful. Often this can be solved by simply asking the doctors if there was a medical reason why your baby was born premie.

Sometimes your behavior or lifestyle could have contributed to the prematurity of your baby. Smoking, drinking and drug abuse are examples. It is best to admit such things, and resolve it. Don't pretend. Rather ask for help. Work through it, deal with it and leave it behind to become healthy for yourself and your baby.

You may be very tired and yet you find it difficult to sleep. When you are tired it is often hard to keep feelings in perspective. The delivery was hard work and worry about your baby's survival and growth also drains your energy. You may find it difficult to concentrate on basic things. Try to get as much rest as possible, and ask for help from friends and family (see page 129).

You may be <u>angry</u> at your situation: "Why me?", "Why was my baby born preterm?" This anger might come out as blaming your partner, or the nurses, or everybody. You may be irritable with your family when they are trying to help.

You may feel <u>very confused</u> by these strong feelings. It is especially important to remember that you have gone through a physical, hormonal and emotional roller-coaster. It takes time to find your balance. <u>Feeling depressed</u> and <u>crying</u> is very common. There is nothing wrong with crying. Tears are deeply healing and release oxytocin, which will calm you.

Some people may use the coping mechanism of being <u>over-optimistic</u>, by <u>denying the reality</u> that there is anything wrong. Be careful of this, as your partner may be in a very different space emotionally.

A preterm birth can cause immense strain on any relationship. Keep talking to each other, with mutual respect and support. Try to understand each other's ways of coping. Sometimes dad has to return to work and can only come to the hospital occasionally. Mom may feel neglected and that he does not care about the baby. Sometimes dad has taken the baby to the NICU, and has had time to learn about the machines and bond with his baby, and then mom feels left out. You may feel upset with the nurses because they are caring for your baby, not you, her mother. You may feel left out. But remember: you are special to your baby, and you are the most important medicine she can get, because only you can give her an emotionally stable environment.

One of the hardest things to cope with is <u>disappointed expectations</u>. This is particularly relevant in modern society where we believe we "should" have control over so many things, health included.

> Every child's life is a gift to receive, not a right to demand.

<u>What can you do to deal with these emotions</u>?

Get involved in caring for your baby (3; 4).

Learn her own unique behavioral cues, the things that make her stressed or relaxed.

Give her as much skin-to-skin contact as you can (5–7).

Find out as much as you can about your baby's condition (we are often afraid of what we don't know).

Ask questions in the NICU.

Ask for help from family.

Talk to other parents of premies in the NICU; they have been in your situation and are often a wonderful support and encouragement.

Talk to a counselor, a social worker or a nurse.

Talk to a caring person. (It is important for dads to do that too.)

Ask for support from Lactation Consultants, and other specialized health professionals.

It may be helpful to make notes of your feelings.

Learn the names of your baby's nurses and doctors. Work with the staff – they are doing all the care and tests <u>for</u> your baby, (not <u>to</u> her!) to help your baby survive.

Allow yourself to cry.

If you have a faith, it may be tested, but it can also be a lifeline.

> Hope is what keeps parents going.

There is a lot you <u>can</u> do to help your tiny new baby even though you may feel helpless because she is so small and frail and fragile and may be linked to so many monitors and machines.

The weeks in NICU may be a roller coaster ride of emotion. Face those feelings.

It may be helpful to make notes of your feelings as this can help you see them more objectively. These strong emotions and worry about your baby's survival can put strain on any loving marriage or relationship. If you are carrying these feelings alone as a single mom or without the loving support of family members it can be very scary and lonely indeed. Worrying whether you have enough money to pay for her care is also difficult. Ask for help!

If your relationship is already strained, the shock of having a premature infant can cause tension between you. However, this can also be an opportunity, a time to work together and draw closer. Keep talking about your feelings to each other, and try to hear each other's emotions without reacting too quickly due to your own pain. Be together. Take time off for a meal or a movie together.

Ideas to help you cope

Your baby may be in the NICU for a long time. You may need to pace yourself for the long haul, so you need to look after yourself.

Get enough sleep. Sleep when your baby sleeps. If necessary, put up a "do not disturb" sign when you are doing skin-to-skin contact.

Eat well. You need to eat healthy snacks to stay healthy. If you get sick, you may not be allowed to visit or hold your baby.

Wear comfortable clothes that button down the front in soft cotton fabrics that will not hurt your baby's skin.

Take a long bath to relax sometimes.

Get outside each day.

Getting exercise will help you keep life in perspective or balance.

Sometimes have family time to be in the NICU together, not just in shifts.

Ask for help from friends and family to look after other children.

Some other things to do:

Have you taken a tiny footprint and handprint of your baby?

Have you taken a weekly picture of your baby? (Do not use a flash which will damage the baby's eyes, rather use a digital camera on a tripod) and watch how quickly she grows.

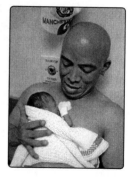

Keep a list of all the specialists that care for your baby. Ask for a primary nurse and doctor. Ask who is the one who makes the decisions about your baby's care.

Record important dates and file information.

Read your baby's chart and ask the staff to explain (write the jargon into the section for this).

Keep a journal for your thoughts. It can be very helpful during the time your baby is in the NICU. Many things will be forgotten, but often writing down the hard thoughts and stages, helps one to see the feelings more objectively. So maybe get a small notebook to keep a record of your feelings. You can also write down questions that you want to ask the doctor when you come in and write down his answers.

Put up photos of your baby.

Enter your baby's unique likes and dislikes on her care plan.

Below is a table to help you, Mom and Dad, to identify the feelings you may experience, but not be able to describe. Circle or mark the ones that speak to you, or write your own over the page. You may need someone to help you do so. Mom and Dad, you have work to do to look after your tiny premature baby and so you need to get to grips with yourselves and your situation as soon as possible in order to help your premature baby effectively.

COMMONLY EXPERIENCED EMOTIONS

Term	Identify from these quotes	Comment	Reason to face issue
Guilt	"What did I do wrong?" "I failed as a mother." "I shouldn't have…"	This is the most common emotion.	You blame yourself so you feel paralyzed.
Inadequacy	"I feel useless here." "I'm redundant, not needed."	This is a totally new situation and you have no clue what to do.	You feel paralyzed.
Incompetence	"What if I do the wrong things?"	You feel disempowered	You do not want to learn the technology.
Helplessness	"I can't do anything for my baby."	You sit blankly.	You feel disempowered.
Denial	"This is not true." "This can't be happening to me." "I don't want this baby."	You have a problem with accepting your baby and your situation. This is often your mind's way of buffering or cushioning the initial shock.	Maybe you do not even want to see your baby in the NICU.

Anger	"Why me?" "My baby was whisked away." "Where has my perfect pregnancy gone?" "This is your fault!"	You feel angry at everything. "Why?"	Blaming others or yourself does not help anyone. You may be angry at your baby for messing up your life and marriage.
Bargaining	"If you save my baby, then I will ...."	You may do this with your spouse or with God.	This is an unrealistic approach.
Depression	"I can't cope any more." "This is hopeless."	When you can no longer deny the reality, the anger may turn inwards to become depression.	Lots of withdrawing or crying can increase the emotional distance between you and your partner and between you and your baby.
Disappointment	"I wanted something else (perfect baby)."		Perhaps you can review your expectations.
Acceptance	"It's going OK."	You have come to terms with your baby's premature birth. Your emotions will have settled.	You are able to keep going through the weeks your baby is in the NICU – this book will give you practical ways to help your baby develop.
Purpose	"We're learning a lot." "I have bonded with my baby."	This is healthy and forward looking	There is a lot you can do practically to help your tiny new baby.

A small note on depression

You may want to withdraw and cry a lot. Do this! Tears are immensely healing and release oxytocin (feel-good hormone), which will make you feel better. It will also help mom to produce breast milk. Exhaustion from not having enough sleep because you are worrying about your premature baby in the NICU can lead to sadness or depression. Here we are looking at mood and emotion, not the clinical condition that needs to be treated with medication. (8)

"Postpartum depression" (PPD) or Postnatal depression (PND) might occur separately. Ask for a professional assessment if the depression goes on for a long time. If you have struggled with depression before, or have a history of depression, it may resurface at this time of worrying about your premature baby. There are simple surveys that you can do to see if you are at risk for PND. The hospital staff can refer you for evaluation and help: there is help for depression! Social workers may want to have a family meeting to try to identify support structures in the home and family and friends that can help the mom and new baby.

Write what emotions you have struggled with. If it is helpful, keep a daily diary or journal of your feelings. Sometimes seeing them on paper helps you cope better and not feel so overwhelmed.

....

....

....

....

....

....

....

....

....

....

....

....

....

....

....

....

....

....

HARD QUESTIONS

Parents of premature babies often have to ask hard questions. Some of these questions do not have easy or immediate answers. It is a very worrying time for parents. It is also concerning for the nurses and doctors who are fighting for your baby's life. You will need to work together and talk through these questions (9).

Some of the early questions:

What are the chances that my baby will survive?

How preterm is she?

Why was she born early?

Whose "fault" is it?

Is it better if she does not survive?

What problems does she have now?

What treatment is she getting?

How can I help my baby in the NICU?

Can I hold her, feed her, etc?

How long does she have to stay in the NICU?

How am I going to cope?

Will I have enough money while my baby is in the NICU?

Questions for the longer term

How will this affect the other siblings and the family?

Will she be able to walk?

Will she be disabled?

Will she need special care later?

Will she develop properly?

Will she be able to attend a normal school?

What are the chances that my baby will survive? (This is always the biggest question that parents of premies face.)

There are no easy answers to this and everything will depend on your baby.

Some important factors

How many weeks preterm was she born? (What is her gestational age?)

What was her birth weight?

Does she have breathing problems?

Does she have birth defects/malformations?

Does she have a disease or infection?

Usually the gestational age is the most important because it will decide if her body organs, particularly her lungs, are developed enough.

Ask your doctor for honest answers. Some babies suddenly get sick and die, others are tiny fighters and keep going even though they have lots of problems.

Survival rates for high-tech NICUs for the USA and Europe:

Less than 21 weeks – no babies will survive

22 weeks – Very few survive

23 weeks   5 – 25%

24 weeks   40 – 60% *   sudden big jump

25 weeks   50 – 80%

26 weeks   80 – 90%

27 weeks   over 90%

* There is a big jump at 24 weeks of gestational age because the lungs are more mature at this point. From 28 weeks, survival in modern NICUs is often very good.

What questions did you have?

....

....

....

....

....

....

....

....

What answers did you receive?

....

....

....

....

....

....

....

....

See the end of this workbook for the different types of support that are available in terms of networks, organizations, people, internet sites and books (see page 145).

Do send your thoughts and experiences for the next edition of this book! This will help another set of parents in this situation!

Send to jill@kangaroomothercare.com

Fine Print Page – Emotions and Coping

1. Bakewell et al provide a framework for comprehensive care that includes specifically aspects related to emotional support to parents.
2. This review identifies and examines common content and processes of postpartum counseling interventions to address trauma symptoms following childbirth. It identifies many of these emotions, while concluding that evidence on how to manage them is lacking!
3. In the past, NICU's discouraged parents from visiting… they and their infants suffered! Parental involvement is essential for subsequent quality outcome.
4. As parents engage, their competence increases, and their contribution to care likewise. They become empowered.
5. Skin-to-Skin Contact is not the focus of this chapter, but SSC does have profound effects on parent's moods, emotions and empowerment.
6. The more parents are involved, and the more SSC they give, the better the bonding and the subsequent developmental outcomes.
7. Tessier elaborates this in a "bonding hypothesis: (KMC) creates a climate in the family whereby parents be-come sensitive care givers. The general hypothesis is that Skin-to-Skin Contact in the KMC group will build up a positive perception in the mothers and a state of readiness to detect and respond to infant's cues."
8. Depression is common and easily overlooked. SSC may directly improve this.
9. This article looks at maternal emotions to low birth weight infants. Quote: "It is possible that among mothers of VLBW infants, for whom none of the oxytocin-releasing conditions were met, oxytocin never reached the level required to activate the development of maternal behavior. Intervention efforts that aim to enhance proximity and touch in VLBW infants, such as skin-to-skin contact , may be crucial for these mothers in order to initiate the bonding process."

Reference List

(1) Bakewell-Sachs S, Gennaro S. Parenting the post-NICU premature infant. MCN The American Journal Of Maternal Child Nursing 2004 November;29(6):398-403.
(2) Gamble J, Creedy D. Content and Processes of Postpartum Counseling After a Distressing Birth Experience: A Review. Birth: Issues in Perinatal Care 2004 September;31(3):213-8.
(3) Latva R, Lehtonen L, Salmelin RK, Tamminen T. Visiting less than every day: a marker for later behavioral problems in Finnish preterm infants. Archives Of Pediatrics & Adolescent Medicine 2004 Decem-ber;158(12):1153-7.
(4) Levy-Shiff R, Sharir H, Mogilner BM. Mother and father preterm infant relationship in the preterm nursery. Child Dev 1989;60(1):93-102.
(5) de Macedo EC, Cruvinel F, Lukasova K, D'Antino ME. The mood variation in mothers of preterm infants in Kangaroo mother care and conventional incubator care. J Trop Pediatr 2007 October 19;53(5):344-6.
(6) Feldman R. Mother-Infant Skin-to-Skin Contact (Kangaroo Care). Infants & Young Children: An Interdisciplinary Journal of Special Care Practices 2004 April;17(2):145-61.
(7) Tessier R, Cristo M, Velez S, Giron M, de Calume ZF, Ruiz-Palaez JG et al. Kangaroo mother care and the bonding hypothesis. Pediatrics 1998 August;102(2):e17 & 390-391.
(8) Dombrowski MA, Anderson GC, Santori C, Burkhammer M. Kangaroo (skin-to-skin) care with a postpartum woman who felt depressed. MCN The American Journal Of Maternal Child Nursing 2001 July;26(4):214-6.
(9) Feldman R, Weller A, Leckman JF, Kuint J, Eidelman AI. The nature of the mother's tie to her infant: mater-nal bonding under conditions of proximity, separation, and potential loss. Journal Of Child Psychology And Psychiatry, And Allied Disciplines 1999 September;40(6):929-39.

SKIN-TO-SKIN CONTACT

Instead of watching your baby in an incubator, keep your naked baby on your chest in skin-to-skin contact. This is the key! It makes the baby:

- feel safe
- become stable
- breastfeed
- brain wire and sleep well
- bond and attach.

Skin-to-Skin Contact is close, direct skin contact between you and your premie. You can be with her for part or all of the day.

HOLD YOUR PREMIE!

How to do Skin-to-Skin Contact

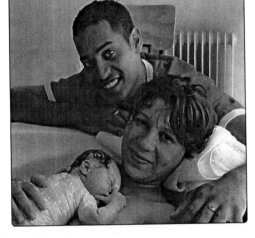

- Place your naked baby onto your bare chest at birth
- She can have on a tiny diaper and a cap if it is very cold
- Cover her with a folded cloth or your shirt
- Talk quietly to her
- When she is sleeping your baby's airway must be secured, and her body supported firmly to your chest

Your body will keep her warm. Your arms will support her and make her feel loved. She feels SAFE with you so her heart rate, blood pressure and oxygen levels stabilize. Emotionally she feels SAFE too. She may even smell her way to Mom's nipple and start to breastfeed.

You have replaced the incubator with your love and care and warmth.

Skin-to-Skin Contact should be given to every full term baby at birth.
It is even more important for fragile premature babies to help them stabilize sooner (4).

When secured safely in Skin-to-Skin Contact with her airway protected, your baby can sleep on your chest as you sleep or walk around.

You can do Skin-to-Skin Contact with your baby on ventilator or other machines.

Your baby will feel SAFE with the familiar sound of your heartbeat, and voice, your warmth and your smell. This feeling of being SAFE helps the baby's heart rate to become even, stable or "regulated." Her blood pressure will be more steady and she will be able to get oxygen around her body properly. As she will feel calmed by your body, her stomach can absorb your breastmilk so she will grow well and healthy. Your body helps stabilize or regulate your baby's body, so she will sooner be able to regulate herself. If she has stress, she can come back to a stable point more quickly.

Her emotional security will also develop better as she feels held, secure, loved and protected so she will bond with you.

Your chest becomes the natural place for growth; she was inside you, but now she can "continue the pregnancy" on your chest. Your body provides her with the warmth, protection and food that she needs for growth, and the security that she needs to wire her brain for healthy relationships.

You (Mom and Dad) become your baby's primary care-givers. The people working in the NICU are there to back you up and support you. You provide warmth, stability, protection. You are forming bonds with your baby which will be the emotional base of her security, which sets a solid base for the rest of her life. We now know that infant mental health leads to adult mental health, so you are giving her the best start.

You are helping your premie to stabilize and her brain to grow best just by being who you are – her mother or her father (the best people to care for her). When you put your tiny baby on your chest, her skin against your skin, she has the right smells, sounds, voice, protection and comfort, (though she may still need the machines for her stability).

Besides helping her to stabilize and her brain to grow, the time spent holding your baby is deeply healing for you and your little premie.

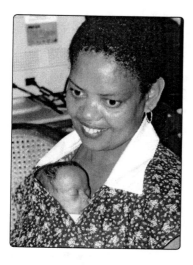
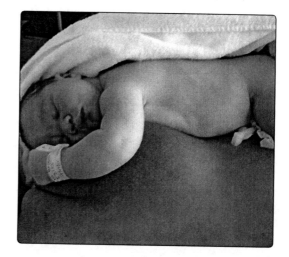

Why carry your baby skin-to-skin?

(Here is the summary, full details follow in this chapter)

Benefits of Skin-to-Skin Contact for babies

> Better brain development
> Better emotional development
> Less stress
> Less crying
> Less brain bleeds
> More settled sleep
> Babies are more alert when they are awake
> Babies feel less pain from injections
> The heart rate stabilizes
> The oxygen saturation is more stable
> Fewer apnea attacks
> Better breathing
> The temperature is most stable on the mother
> Breastfeeding starts more easily
> More breastmilk is produced
> Gestation-specific milk is produced.
> Faster weight gain
> Baby can usually go home earlier

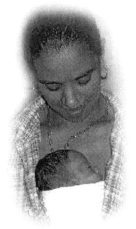

Benefits of Skin-to-Skin Contact for parents

> Parents become central to the caring team
> Better bonding and interaction with their child
> Emotional healing
> Less guilt feelings and other negative emotions
> Parents are calmer
> Parents are empowered and more confident
> Parents are able to learn their baby's unique cues for hunger
> Parents and baby get more sleep
> Parents (especially mothers), are less depressed
> Parents cope better in NICU
> Parents see baby as less "abnormal"

1 How to do Skin-to-Skin Contact when your baby is born

Your baby can lie on your tummy straight after birth. Here she can be dried by being wiped gently and covered with a cloth. When the cord stops pulsating it can be cut.

Mom, take off your bra but keep your shirt on; it is easiest if you have one that buttons down the front. Now baby can be placed on your chest, against your skin.

Lie a little upright, a 30-40 degree angle helps her breathing. Leave her hands free, and allow her head movements. You can hold your hands underneath and behind her.

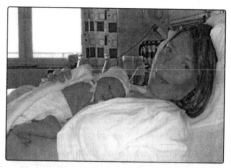

Cover yourself and your premie. Your body will automatically warm up if your baby is cold, or will cool down if your baby is hot. You might find that you start to sweat; don't worry, that is normal.

If it is cold in the room, you may want to put a small hat on her head, as most of the body heat is lost through the head. For a tiny baby, losing heat means that she uses lots of calories that she should be using to grow. Make sure that all materials are pure cotton as her skin is extremely sensitive. When convenient, put the diaper on. Turn down the lights.

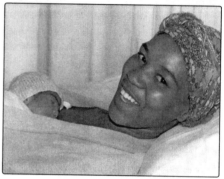

Keep this position for the next hour or so, and just watch while your baby finds her way in her new world!

Do not interrupt this early behavior!

Note: For the first hour after birth, your baby's biology wants her to be free to crawl to your breast, so she should be loose (1). After the first hour, and if you want to sleep, her airway needs to be secured.

2 How to do Skin-to-Skin Contact after the first hour

For the first six hours in Skin-to-Skin Contact, your premie is stabilizing her heart and lungs. During this time it is best to sit or lie down, leaning at an angle (30-40 degrees).

One very important thing to know: your premie baby does not have neck control, and we want to prevent "obstructive apnea" – a closed airway that stops her breathing. To secure her airway, place her on your chest as above. Her head should be turned to the side and tilted slightly up (sniffing position), so that her airway is open fully. Take a fine weave cotton wrap and fold it under her chin and ear and around your back so she is tied firmly over your chest bone (2). This will fix her airway to your chest, and at the same time secure her to your body. Importantly, the wrap must not be made with stretch material as it will not keep the airway open safely. Now, using your shirt or a longer cloth, secure the rest of her body to yours (see page 49 how the KangaCarrier or the "Thari" does this).

This will free your arms so that you can relax, read etc, but also be able to keep this up for long periods. Always aim at giving skin-to-skin for at least one full hour.

Your baby can be held in Skin-to-Skin Contact as long as you want, for part or all of 24 hours a day. To get the full benefits of Skin-to-Skin Contact, it is important for your baby to go through at least a full sleep-wake cycle which is usually about 60 minutes to get her biological systems stabilized. A tiny premie's body systems will not be mature enough for her to stabilize herself, and mother's chest will help her to settle in to a sleep-cycling and breastfeeding rhythm.

All of this can be done by dad if mom has had a caesarean section. It can be done in Labor ward, post natal ward or neonatal Unit.

3 How to do Skin-to-Skin Contact after six hours

You can start Skin-to-skin contact at any time! When you do this for the first time, tell your baby what you are going to do. Undress her, turn her over on to her front before you pick her up, and then place her gently on your naked chest. Your nurse can help you until you can do this yourself. As described above, secure the baby's neck and head against your chest with a wrap-around non-stretch cotton cloth. Her face should be looking up, and her head close enough to kiss. Then cover both of you with a shirt that

supports and contains the baby's body against your own. Your baby will in most cases settle down to sleep straight away. Keep this position when sleeping.

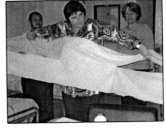

A thari wrap

With your baby in skin-to-skin contact you will be able to feel if she is asleep or awake. This is very valuable and very important, as NICU's usually don't have monitors that can tell this. But you will be able to tell not just if baby is sleeping but how deeply. When your baby is in the deepest part of sleep, brain wiring is taking place (see page 83). So you can work with the nursing staff to protect the sleep cycle of your baby, and delay non-urgent treatment until baby wakes.

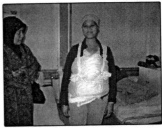

You may cry with relief as you hold her – that is normal. You will feel full of wonder to be able to hold your tiny baby, knowing that you are giving her the best, just by being her mother or her father. Tears are deeply healing. Mom, you will release oxytocin which will make you calmer and therefore your baby calmer too. Your tears will also help your milk production. Dad, you can cry too. You might feel fearful as your tiny premie seems so very fragile.

When your baby wakes up, untie the wrap, and the shirt, and let her slide down onto your breast, still in skin-to-skin contact. Here she is in the right place to breastfeed, and she will do so without any help.

4 How to do Skin-to-Skin Contact with a very small baby (even with technology)

You may only be able to start skin-to-skin contact some time after birth. This can all be done with the technology that the very small premie requires. Start doing this as soon as it is possible. Begin by making yourself comfortable in a chair, ideally one that can recline. Moving the baby requires making sure there is enough length of cables and tubing, and then these can be secured to your skin or your shirt with tape. Tie the baby

The KangaCarrier helps you to do skin-to-skin <u>all</u> the time

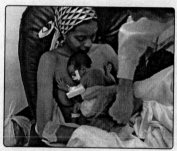

Place baby in Skin-to-Skin Contact on mother's chest bone, hands near her mouth, arms bent, legs bent (flexed).

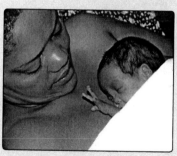

Tie baby on tightly under chin and ear with white cloth, to fix airway.

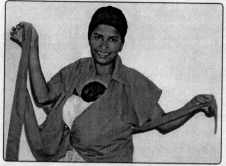

Mother puts on KangaCarrier shirt, the first wraparound should fit tightly under baby's bottom, and include the legs.

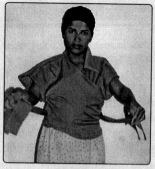

Put second wraparound as overlap and tie firmly.

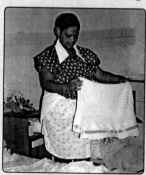

Baby is fully contained and feels safe, mother can use both hands and walk around freely.

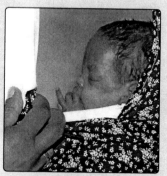

Baby can sleep comfortably.

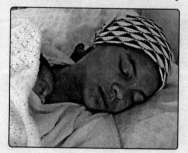

Mother can also sleep with baby safe.

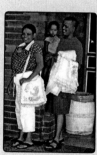

Mother can go home 'wearing' her premie

to your chest as above. The smaller the baby is, the more close and tight she needs to be fastened.

The staff will give you advice and help, and are there to support you and teach you according to the specific needs of your baby. The nurses will help you to transfer her to your chest, especially if she needs respirators, monitors, etc. The nurses might tape the cables and tubes together to make it easier to work with them.

> **The smaller the premie, the more she needs her mother's chest to stabilize even if she needs medical technology as well. (4)**

You give closeness and security to your child. Positive feelings for your child strengthen as you care for your baby and closeness helps you to interpret your baby's unique small signals. For example, you will know very quickly when she is ready to breastfeed, is tired or stressed. Being held skin-to-skin, contained and secure is the best thing for your premie's physical, mental and emotional health.

5 Skin-to-skin contact and walking around

When your premie is stable enough, it may be more comfortable for you to get up and move around holding her in Skin-to-Skin Contact (the Kangaroo Position). The KangaCarrier or Thari mentioned above make this possible. If monitors are connected to her, keep them on while you stand up the first time to confirm her stability. If she is connected to machines, you can only move as far as the leads allow.

Soon, you will be able to get up and move around more freely with your baby tied to your chest. You can read or write, talk to friends and even make tea or a meal.

6 Skin-to-skin contact and sleeping

You can sleep with your premie in skin-to-skin, as long as her airway is stabilized and she is held safely in the wrap. You can lie on your back or on your side with your head slightly raised. Your baby is used to being held tightly in the womb and feels safer when she is contained. The doctor will decide if your premie needs technical monitoring while she is sleeping.

> **A baby in quiet sleep should never be disturbed**

When your premie starts to wake up or wriggle, you can loosen the tie and feed her. Change her diaper if needed, and spend time looking at her and talking to her. When she is awake, the nurses can do the tests they need to do. After that, tie her on firmly again so that she can sleep.

> **Remember that it is important for your baby to go through at least a full sleep-wake cycle (usually about 60-90 minutes) to get the full benefits of Skin-to-Skin Contact and for brain wiring (3).**

Mom and Dad, you can take it in turns to hold your child in Skin-to-Skin Contact. If you have twins, Dad, granny, aunt, or close friend can carry one twin skin-to-skin while Mom holds the other. For best effects before breastfeeding it would need to be Mom who holds the baby. If you want to hold your premie in continuous Skin-to-Skin Contact, it will also work to ask a relative or close friend to take turns in holding her in Skin-to-Skin Contact.

> **Important:** If you need to leave the ward, your premie can be left warmly wrapped in a bed <u>only</u> if she is able to maintain a stable body temperature on her own. Below 4 lb, an infant needs to be warmed as she cannot do this for herself.

When to do Skin-to-Skin Contact (SSC)

Whenever you possibly can!

Skin-to-Skin Contact should be given to every baby at birth.
It is even more important for premature babies to help them stabilize (4).
You can do Skin-to-Skin Contact when you are sleeping, or walking around.
You can do Skin-to-Skin Contact with a baby on a ventilator or other machines (5).

Some situations allow Skin-to-Skin Contact or "Kangaroo Care" only as an add-on to incubator care, or as a bit of cuddling for 10-60 minutes a day. This helps mom and baby to bond together and does help the mother produce more breastmilk (6)! However, if you hold your baby for less than an hour, or less than one full sleep-awake cycle, it may be of no benefit to her brain (7).

Skin-to-Skin Contact should ideally be 24 hours a day so that your baby is never separated from you, her Mom (8). More realistic is for mom and dad to take it in turns for the full 24 hours! In this way, her stress levels are kept as low as possible. Some hospitals do not have enough space for parents to sleep in the hospital, but now that you know how important it is that her brain wires properly, you will make it a priority to spend as much time as possible with her (9).

Take leave, get home help or do whatever is needed to give your premie your support – she is fighting for her life and she needs you to help her. You will never regret this time that you spend with her.

Can you still do Skin-to-Skin Contact when your baby is jaundiced?

Hospitals have routinely left babies in incubators under ultraviolet light to correct their bilirubin levels if they look "yellow." This is needed for the baby but is often a lonely and worrying time for the parents who are told that they cannot hold their baby. There are ways to change this. Some places have bilirubin blankets so that the baby can be on mother and get the ultraviolet from a pad on her back. Other places can put dark covers over baby's eyes, and give baby ultraviolet treatment on mom's chest, with both under the lights. If we understand the importance of not separating mom and baby there can always be creative solutions.

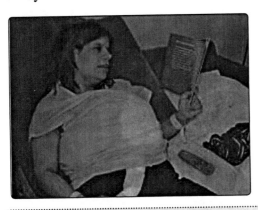

Babies getting phototherapy on mom.

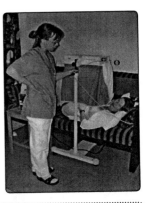

....
The smaller the prem, the more she needs her mother's chest to stabilise even if she needs medical technology as well. (See fine print page reference 4)
....

Details of the benefits of Skin-to-Skin Contact

<u>**There are many benefits for the baby.**</u>

Babies stabilize faster when cared for in Skin-to-Skin Contact than in incubators (See Ref (4) - Babies do not stabilize as well in the incubator in the first six hours of

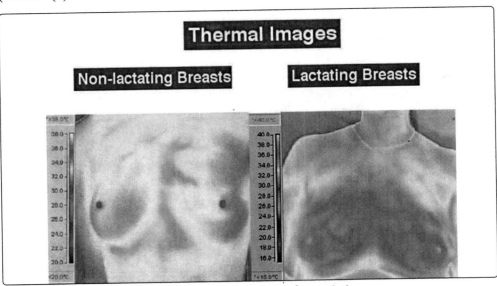

Ref: Peter Hartmann, used with permission.

life). Contact with a parent's skin helps the baby to maintain a more even temperature, heart rate, oxygen saturation and metabolism (10). The temperature on the chest of a breastfeeding mother is about 3°F higher than that of a non-lactating mother (11). The mother's core temperature will automatically rise to warm a cold infant and drop to cool a hot infant. Studies have shown that the two breast temperatures can act independently with twins of different temperatures! (12) Adjustment to life outside the womb is one of the most challenging times of change, and this is made safer by Skin-to-Skin Contact. The benefits are faster weight gain and better quiet sleep when the main growth occurs (3), without the baby going into too deep sleep level. Fewer stress hormones are released in connection with the handling necessary for care. These stress hormones contribute to brain bleeds in premature infants.

Breastmilk production The babies are stimulated to breastfeed as they can smell the mothers' milk. The Skin-to-Skin Contact between mother and baby stimulates prolactin and oxytocin production which increases milk production (13).

The baby gets all the benefits of breastmilk, including the correct milk for humans. (Formula is made with cows' milk which is designed for baby calves. The main protein in cows' milk, casein, is toxic to the human baby's gut, and may lead to milk allergies on formula.)

The babies can breastfeed more often in Skin-to-Skin Contact (SSC) as it encourages frequent feeding. This is helpful for growth as the premie baby's stomach is very small at birth. The baby smells the breastmilk straight away so the rooting instinct clicks in quickly and there are fewer problems with breastfeeding later. When the baby latches on to the breast correctly, there is less breast engorgement and the mother's nipples are not as sore. If the baby is preterm she also gets gestation-specific breastmilk. The milk content varies according to the baby's needs. The breastmilk contains all the ingredients necessary for brain growth.

> **In terms of protection, there will be fewer infections as the mom in the NICU will produce antibodies to the natural bacteria in the NICU and pass these antibodies onto her baby through the breastmilk (14). The baby will get antibodies and about a thousand other protective factors from her mother's milk. The mother's colostrum carries the antibodies needed to protect the newborn with immunity. There are fewer long-term health problems for babies that have breastfed and had Skin-to-Skin Contact; there are also fewer allergies (15).**

Faster growth: In Skin-to-Skin Contact, the baby is in a relaxed mode so all her hormones prepare her gut to absorb food maximally. Babies in Skin-to-Skin Contact can grow at 1 oz per day which is twice the rate of an incubator baby (2). Skin-to-Skin Contact can mean less time in hospital (16).

A major benefit of skin-to-skin contact is that the babies cry less so they have less stress hormones circulating (e.g. somatostatin and high levels of cortisol) (17). Somatostatin shuts down the gut and slows growth. Cortisol increases blood pressure and contributes to brain bleeds which are very common in premature infants.

In Skin-to-Skin Contact, the development of the baby is the best. The baby is in the right place and therefore has the right behavior. Skin-to-Skin Contact helps the baby to self-regulate and organize her systems. Without the presence of mother, the baby cannot bring her stress hormones down or get her brain to produce oxytocin to relax herself. The physical contact of co-sleeping or skin-to skin contact helps the baby to regulate her brain's stress response system (18).

The small movements of her mother's chest and hearing her heartbeat remind the baby to breathe so there is less apnea.

<u>Bonding:</u> The baby is emotionally secure in Skin-to-Skin Contact and the mother-infant bond is established early. This will mean that the baby will have better long term <u>emotional stability</u>. The primary bond of mother and child is the base on which all later relationships are built. There is increased intimacy and attachment and eye contact between mom and baby (19). Skin-to-skin contact is especially good for mothers who experience difficult births or postnatal depression, also for fathers and adoptive parents.

<u>The developmental pathways of the brain</u> grow best without stress. Learning is helped because of periods of quiet awareness. Rapid eye movement (REM) and non-REM sleep are both needed for memory formation. (See page 83, the section on protecting sleep).

Skin-to-Skin Contact has many benefits for you as her mother.

Skin–to-Skin Contact at birth helps you to bond with your baby immediately; it also releases oxytocin making you calmer, and prolactin to start the production of breastmilk.

> **When a baby is born too early, the mother often feels helpless. Holding your baby in Skin-to-Skin Contact will empower you to be part of the caring team and feel that you are able to really help your baby.**
>
> **When you are close to your tiny baby, you will feel calmer (both parents); Skin-to-Skin Contact allows you to give closeness and security to your child. Positive feelings for your baby strengthen as you care for her, and closeness helps you to interpret your baby's small signals, for example when she is waking up and ready to breastfeed.**

Breastfeeding releases hormones which help to contract mum's uterus, resulting in less blood loss right after delivery. The Skin-to-Skin Contact helps you and your baby to settle into a rhythm of sleeping and waking together – "sleep synchrony" – so you both actually get more sleep.

Feelings of trauma at her early birth or the feelings of guilt at not carrying your baby to full term are eased by Skin-to-Skin Contact. Mothers often have a sense of guilt and anxiety when they deliver their babies preterm and are prone to post-partum depression. Holding your baby on your chest in Skin-to-Skin Contact helps you to feel that she is completing her gestation and that you are giving her the best possible care.

Carrying your premie in Skin-to-Skin Contact means that you are able to be mobile sooner and can leave the hospital earlier. You will also be able to return to normal daily life sooner. (Having your baby secured firmly and safely on your chest in Skin-to-Skin Contact will make a huge difference when you get home as you can do chores while still giving your baby the best care.)

Observing the benefits of skin to skin contact

For your baby	Date first seen
Her heart rate stabilizes sooner	
Her oxygen saturation improves	
Her temperature is more stable	
She cries less	
She seems more peaceful	
She sleeps better	
She has less apnea attacks	
She has been able to start breastfeeding	
She grows faster on the days she has more skin to skin contact.	

For mom	
You feel more peaceful and calm carrying your baby	
You feel a closer bond to your baby	
You can sleep when your baby sleeps	
You get more sleep	
You can read her tiny stress cues more easily	
You can breastfeed more easily	
You feel empowered and competent to care for your baby	
You feel less fearful or guilty	
You seem to have more breastmilk	
You feel more normal, and less like a patient	
You feel that you can cope better	
You feel more hopeful for the future	

Fine Print Page – Skin-to-Skin Contact

This chapter addresses SSC for the parent: the references here support the statements and claims made. It is a long chapter, and so there are two fine print pages !!!!

1. Righard describes the natural birth behavior, available as a video from www.geddesproduction.com . This research is also described by Widstrom (1987)
2. The KangaCarrier technique described in this chapter was developed and tested in a situation without incuba-tors, by both authors and midwife Agneta Jurisoo, and provides safe 24 hour care. It was also tested in a RCT, see below. It frees mother's arms so as to allow safe sleep and also being able to stand and walk, within limits of IV lines and monitoring equipment.
3. The importance of sleep cycling is one of the key findings of recent neuroscience, and this paper describes the effect on SSC on sleep cycling. The advice given here is based on this.
4. The RCT by Bergman, Linley and Fawcus looked directly at comparing stabilization. ALL babies 1200g to 2200g stabilized by 6 hours in SSC, only half those in incubators, the smaller the babies were, the more un-stable they were in the incubator. Approximately 200 trials comparing SSC and incubator have all shown SSC to be as good or better ... but because incubator is still assumed to be normal, SSC is now merely ac-cepted. Actually, both from biology and neuroscience, SSC is normal, and the separation of the incubator makes the baby worse, it dys-regulates the normal physiology.
5. Having said that SSC is better than incubator, very small babies still need the technology that supports imma-ture respiratory function! None of the technology currently used in intensive care units is a contraindication to doing SSC. Obviously, SSC must be practiced safely and with experience, and with due protocol. This pa-per describes some specific issues in doing so. Where experience is lacking and equipment unsuitable, SSC may not be advis-able. A number of medical complications (e.g. gastroschisis, meningomyelocele) may also make SSC ill-advised.
6. In this rather old study, mothers did only 10 minutes of SSC a day, and yet it almost doubled their milk pro-duction. SSC allows increased suckling opportunity with hormones improving milk production, and en-hances relaxation and parasympathetic stimulation.
7. Short periods may be good for mom, but not for baby. This study giving 20 min of SSC for extreme low birth weight babies "showed neither benefit or harm", and the authors do not recommend the "extra trouble and re-sources required". 20 minutes is too little!! Less than one sleep cycle does not allow for a sleep cycle, and is not recommended! There are a few other studies with similar results.
8. The "Kangaroo Mother Care" as defined by the World Health Organisation (WHO) advises continuous SSC, starting as early as possible, and also includes exclusive breastfeeding.
9. The WHO guide also provides practical guidelines for implementing and practicing SSC.
10. This article summarizes much of the broader aspects of the physiological benefits.
11. The higher skin temperature means this is the biological extra-uterine habitat for newborns
12. Mother's chest controls infant temperature in a narrow and stable range.
13. Uvnas-Moberg provides a review of the hormonal effects, includes pacifier effects.
14. In this careful prospective study, being fed infant formula increased infections from 29% (mother's milk fed) to 47%, and serious infections increased likewise: 19.5% vs 32.6%.
15. This recent WHO report provides the latest evidence on benefits, it is now firmly established that breastfeed-ing and mother's milk are superior, and formula is harmful.
16. In this study, premature babies got just 2 hours SSC starting when they were 3lbs 5oz, they grew 0,10 oz a day faster, and they went home two days earlier.
17. This second article discussing somatostatin makes more direct links to SSC.
18. These comments are based on an interpretation of Schore's work, and other researchers (Teicher, Perry), and extrapolated in ongoing research to newborns.
19. Klaus and Kennell's work on "bonding" was discredited at the time, but is in fact supported by the most recent neuroscience.
20. Finally, here is the first review on KC, which is still valid, by Anderson (20).
21. The latest Cochrane review, updated 2008 (21).

There about 200 studies looking at specific outcomes, (temperature, heart rate, oxygen saturation etc), and Susan Ludington in Cleveland keeps an up to date inventory of these, older versions are available on www.kangaroomothercare.com

Reference List

(1) Righard L, Alade MO. Effect of delivery room routines on success of first breast-feed. Lancet 1990 November 3;336(8723):1105-7.
(2) Bergman NJ, Jurisoo LA. The 'kangaroo-method' for treating low birth weight babies in a developing coun-try. Trop Doct 1994 April;24(2):57-60.
(3) Ludington-Hoe Sm, Johnson MW, Morgan K, Lewis T, Gutman J, Wilson D et al. Neurophysiologic assess-ment

of neonatal sleep organization: Preliminary results of a randomized, controlled trial of skin contant with preterm infants. Pediatrics 2006 May;112(5):e909-e923.

(4)   Bergman NJ, Linley LL, Fawcus SR. Randomized controlled trial of Skin-to-Skin Contact from birth versus conventional incubator for physiological stabilization in 1200- to 2199-gram newborns. Acta Paediatr 2004 June;93(6):779-85.

(5)   Ludington-Hoe Sm, FC, SJ, .Ceccardi JJ. Safe Criteria and Procedure for Kangaroo Care with Intubated Preterm Infants. JOGNN: Journal of Obstetric, Gynecologic, & Neonatal Nursing 2003 Septem-ber;32(5):579-88.

(6)   Hurst NM, Valentine CJ, Renfro L, Burns P, Ferlic L. Skin-to-skin holding in the neonatal intensive care unit influences maternal milk volume. J Perinatol 1997 May;17(3):213-7.

(7)   Miles R, Cowan F, Glover V, Stevenson J, Modi N. A controlled trial of Skin-to-Skin Contact in extremely pre-term infants. Early Human Development 2006 July;82(7):447-55.

(8)   Cattaneo A, Davanzo R, Bergman N, Charpak N. Kangaroo mother care in low-income countries. Interna-tional Network in Kangaroo Mother Care. J Trop Pediatr 1998 October;44(5):279-82.

(9)   WHO. Kangaroo mother care - a practical guide. WHO; 2003.

(10)   Ludington-Hoe SM, Swinth JY. Developmental aspects of kangaroo care. J Obstet Gynecol Neonatal Nurs 1996 October;25(8):691-703.

(11)   Bauer K, Pasel K, Versmold H. Chest skin temperature of mothers of term and preterm infants is higher than that of men and women. Pediatric Research 39[4], part2-195A. 1996.
        Ref Type: Journal (Full)

(12)   Ludington-Hoe Sm, Lewis T, Morgan K, Cong X, Anderson L, Reese S. Breast-infant temperature synchrony with twins during shared kangaroo care. JOGNN 2006;35(2):1-9.

(13)   Uvnas-Moberg K, Eriksson M. Breastfeeding: physiological, endocrine and behavioural adaptations caused by oxytocin and local neurogenic activity in the nipple and mammary gland. Acta Paediatr 1996 May;85(5):525-30.

(14)   Hylander MA, Strobino DM, Dhanireddy R. Human milk feedings and infection among very low birth weight infants. Pediatrics 1998 September;102(3):E38.

(15)   WHO. Systematic reviews: Evidence on the long-term effects of breastfeeding. WHO 2007.

(16)   Hann M, Malan A, Kronson M, Bergman N, Huskisson J. Kangaroo mother care. S Afr Med J 1999 Janu-ary;89(1):37-9.

(17)   Uvnas-Moberg K, Widstrom AM, Marchini G, Winberg J. Release of GI hormones in mother and infant by sen-sory stimulation. Acta Paediatr Scand 1987 November;76(6):851-60.

(18)   Schore AN. Dysregulation of the right brain: a fundamental mechanism of traumatic attachment and the psycho-pathogenesis of posttraumatic stress disorder. Aust N Z J Psychiatry 2002 February;36(1):9-30.

(19)   Klaus MH, Kennell JH. Maternal infant bonding. St Louis MO: CV Mosby; 1976.

(20)   Anderson GC. An overview of research data and descriptive reports in the English language on kangaroo care, 1983- 1991. Journal of Perinatology X1[3], 218-226. 1991.
        Ref Type: Magazine Article

(21)   Moore ER, Anderson GC, Bergman N. Early Skin-to-Skin Contact for mothers and their healthy newborn infants. Cochrane Database of Systematic Reviews 2008;(4).

BREASTMILK AND BREASTFEEDING

> **Mom, do ALL you possibly can to express milk for your preterm baby.**
> **No one else can do this for her.**

This chapter has three sections:

1   <u>Breastmilk</u> (see page 59)
- [ ] is the right food for your baby's brain to grow.
- [ ] Your premie needs breastmilk even more than a full term baby.
- [ ] Your baby needs colostrum to protect her gut.
- [ ] has FAR more benefits than formula.
- [ ] is dynamic; produced for your specific baby at her specific stage of development.

2   <u>Ways of feeding premies</u> (see page 65)
- [ ] By TPN (Total Parenteral nutrition, ie intravenous feeding)
- [ ] By NGT or OGT (naso- or oro-gastric tube)
- [ ] By cup
- [ ] By breastfeeding

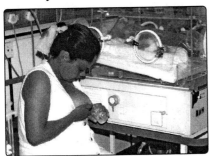
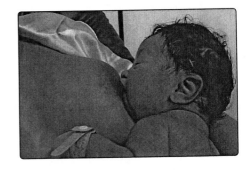

3   <u>Breastfeeding your premie</u> (see page 72)
- [ ] "Breastfeeding is normal".
- [ ] Breastfeeding provides the right sensations for brain-wiring.
- [ ] If you want to breastfeed, start expressing straight away.
- [ ] When you hold your baby in Skin-to-Skin Contact, you produce more breastmilk.
- [ ] The more often your baby feeds, the more breast milk is produced.
- [ ] From 28 weeks gestation onwards, a premie is able to suckle on the breast.

> **Breastfed is normal, accept no substitutes.**

The stomach of a prem is tiny, so she will prefer to be fed small amounts often (every 60-90 minutes).

Bottle feeding is stressful for a baby.

1 BREASTMILK

> **Firstly: your baby's brain needs the correct food: breastmilk.**

This section is valid for ALL babies. Later we will focus specifically on premature babies.

Look at this list of amazing benefits of breastmilk and you will see why it is so important to give your baby your breastmilk (1). It is one of the most important things that you as a mother can do for your baby, to give her health now and in the future.

MORE BENEFITS

Breastmilk:

- is the best food for overall growth, especially for brain growth.
- has antibodies to protect against and to fight infections.
- changes to meet the baby's specific needs over time.
- gives better bone density.

FEWER PROBLEMS

Feeding breastmilk reduces:

- sickness and time in hospital;
- diarrhea and vomiting;
- infection of the gut (gastroenteritis);
- necrotizing enterocolitis (NEC, a nasty kind of gut infection);
- colic;
- childhood diabetes or obesity;
- ear infections;
- respiratory infections (pneumonia, bronchitis etc);
- allergies, less asthma;
- blood poisoning (septicemia);
- Sudden Infant Death Syndrome (SIDS, cot death);
- meningitis;
- tooth decay;
- risk of heart disease later in life;
- risk of Vitamin D and iron deficiencies.

What milk? Breastmilk!

Humans are "mammals", and in biological terms being a mammal means that we breastfeed our babies our own unique milk. The "Professional Advice" that tells mothers not to exclusively breastfeed is not based on science! There is now overwhelming evidence that mother's own milk is the best food for babies (see fine print page) (1;2).

> Mom: make <u>every effort</u> to get your own milk to your baby, it is vital.

Breastmilk changes throughout the tiny baby's life and is different from birth to a week, to a month, to a year. **Breastmilk is dynamic; it is produced for that specific baby at that specific stage of development.** It will be thinner if it is hot and the baby many need extra fluids. It changes through the day (3).

You may have heard the slogan, "Breast is best". This implies that formula is OK.

> "Breastfeeding is normal" is more accurate.

Putting it this way tells you that anything else is abnormal, and therefore worse! Your baby needs normal good food, not abnormal replacement. Breastmilk is the only right milk for the human baby. It has over a thousand different components which the baby needs (4). Formula has only 30! All formula companies know that breastmilk is the "gold standard", and try to copy it. That should tell you just how valuable breast milk is! Formula can never be as good as breastmilk. Artificial formula comes from cows that produce milk designed for calves that eat grass and have four stomachs.

Formula is abnormal for human babies. It has even been suggested that formula should only be allowed on prescription!

Two thirds of mother's milk protein is whey which contains antibodies and immune protection factors. Most of cow's milk is casein, and cow casein is very different from human casein. When cow casein breaks down it makes compounds that can damage the human baby's gut (maybe this is why formula-fed babies get colic). This is even more of a problem for a premature, whose gut is more sensitive.

Human milk is 25% NPN, (non-protein nitrogen) (3); these are 200 or more different tiny proteins ready for building the human baby's brain and gut, and providing immune protection. Cow's milk has only 2% of these NPNs! .

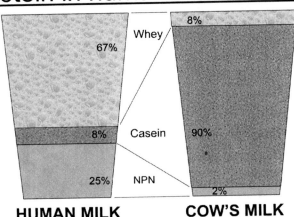

Protein in human and cow milk

HUMAN MILK — Whey 67%, 8%, 25%
COW'S MILK — 8%, Casein 90%, NPN 2%

HUMAN MILK   **COW'S MILK**

Breastmilk and prematurity

So – is this information on breastmilk relevant for your PRETERM baby? Absolutely! (6)

> **Premie babies need breastmilk even more than full-term babies.**

Premies are often unable to keep their fluid balance right. Premies dry out very quickly through their very thin skin and through their lungs. Their bodies are 90% water, so one of the big challenges is to get enough fluid into your baby, and also to get enough food, not just for survival, but to actively grow.

Your tiny premie may desperately need the fluids and nutrition while your breastmilk is starting so the NICU staff may give her other food. Total Parenteral Nutrition (TPN) is often given intravenously, as a temporary measure until you can give breastmilk. (I will say a little more in the next section, see page 65.)

The first breastmilk produced looks very different but it is VERY important to give this "colostrum" to the baby as soon after birth as possible. Colostrum has surface antibodies that protect the stomach lining, as well as a lot of other protective factors. Even three drops can help! That is why it is called "liquid gold".

> **Every baby needs colostrum to protect the gut.**
> **Even one "top up" feed of formula will disturb the gut of the newborn for life!**

Formula fed premies have a 6–9 times increase in necrotizing enterocolitis (NEC), a severe gut infection premies may get. The baby's metabolism will adapt better if she is breastfed, than if she is artificially fed. It is also better if she is exclusively breastfed than if she has mixed feeds (getting some breastmilk, some formula) (8).

Breastmilk contains long- and medium-chain fatty acids (called omega 6 and 3). These fats make myelin, which coats the nerves and acts a bit like insulation around an electric cord. This makes sending messages in the brain faster, an important part of future intelligence (9). It is correct to say that breastmilk increases intelligence! (10) Nothing else can do this for the brain. Interestingly, the fat content of the mother's milk increases over the first year, when more myelin is needed in the brain. (11)

> **Any amount of your breastmilk that you can supply to your baby is important, specifically for her brain growth.**
> **Babies need only breastmilk for brain growth.**

The baby's brain is the most important organ being developed in the last ten weeks of pregnancy. If the baby is born too early, the mother's body automatically produces in her breastmilk what her premie baby would have received via the umbilical cord and what she needs for her brain to grow properly. Mother's milk is "gestation–specific". That is, the food in the breastmilk of a 27 week gestation baby is different from the food for a baby of 31 weeks gestation, which is different from the food for a full term baby. The contents of the milk are different for each breastfeeding premature baby to supply the individual needs of that specific baby at that time.

Expressing breastmilk

The next important thing is how to get this milk!

> **Almost every mother is able to produce breastmilk.**

It is important to express milk because you are providing your baby with the best nutrition; nutrition that no-one else can duplicate at a critical time in her life. It may take extra time and hard work to express milk, but as you have read – it is well worth the effort. Breastmilk is the best food for your baby's brain. You may want to invest in the help of a supportive lactation consultant to help get your milk production going – it is really worthwhile (6).

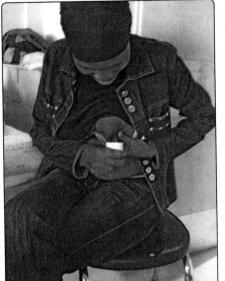

Hand expressing

If your baby has delivered normally, your body will have started producing hormones like prolactin to start the production of milk, and oxytocin to release it. Skin-to-Skin Contact aids the release of these hormones, which is another reason why it is so essential!!

Start expressing milk at birth or within 6 hours. Remember that those first few drops of colostrum are important to protect your baby's stomach. You can express your breastmilk by hand or you can use a pump to get your milk going. If you are using a pump, start on the lowest setting for 5 minutes a side every 2–3 hours during the day and 3–4 hourly at night. It is better to pump often and for short times to get the milk started. By the second day you can pump for 10 minutes at a time. You may feel anxious that you have to produce enough milk, but your baby needs less in the first few days. It will be easier to pump milk if you can see or touch your baby while pumping. Your milk will increase in volume the more you pump and by two weeks you should aim for at least 18 fl oz (500ml) per day, the more the better. This is more than your baby needs now, but this volume cannot easily be increased after the first few weeks. You can store the excess, or donate to a milk bank (to help another mom who may be struggling.) If you have sore or cracked nipples, spread breastmilk on them regularly and let them dry in fresh air. No cream is needed.

> **If you do want to breastfeed, start expressing straight away.**

If you hold your baby in Skin-to-Skin Contact, more milk will be produced, your baby will be calmer, and should latch better. Carry her skin-to-skin for 15 to 30 minutes before a feed. This will calm you and your baby! Hormones are released in your baby to prepare her gut to receive the milk. At the same time the hormones work in you to produce and let the milk flow down.

Follow your hospital guidelines for milk storage. As a general rule, Expressed Breastmilk (EBM) can be safely stored for

- 4 hours in a cool room;
- 24 hours in a fridge (<39°F);
- 2 weeks in a freezer compartment;
- 3 months in a freezer.

Important: This milk needs to be carefully labeled with your name and the date and time

> **If you read this before giving birth, plan to give your baby colostrum.**
> **Express milk for your baby as soon after birth as you can.**
> **Express milk as frequently as possible.**
> **Keep expressing to get your milk flowing**

it was expressed.

For moms

It is normal to produce small amounts during the first few days. Your baby needs these few drops at a time in the first few days.

How much milk could you produce   first day? ....

second day? ....

third day ? ....

end of week 1 ....

end of week 2

Now that we know that it is essential to give your premie breastmilk, let us look at how to get it into her!

> **If for any reason you cannot or should not breastfeed, then give your baby extra Skin-to-Skin Contact. !! This way she will get the sensory and social benefits that her brain needs for its development.**

Fine Print Page – Breastmilk and Breastfeeding

There are more breastfeeding references in the next two chapters!

1. Policy statement from American Academy of Pediatrics updated recommendations on breastfeeding, summarizes evidence at 2005, which has increased since then.
2. World Health Organization systematic review on long term effects, shows breastfeeding improves blood pressure, cholesterol, overweight, schooling and IQ.
3. Milk volume is shown to be directly determined by infant demand, other factors also, see also ref 5.
4. There are a whole variety of different immune systems and mechanisms, and they act synergistically. One single group alone, the glycans, has several thousand different varieties.
5. This article highlights differences between human and cows milk in all aspects. (For more on NPN see Rudloff & Kunz 1997).
6. This article summarizes benefits specific to premature infants, and then gives general advice on how to ensure feeding by mothers' own milk can be adopted by neonatal units.
7. Reviews development of the gut in relation to colostrum, there are other functions of colostrum also! Dr Sears writes that one drop of milk contains one million active immunity cells.
8. Exclusive really means nothing else … complementary feeding is harmful.
9. One single gene, FADS2, will make for a 6 – 8 point increase in IQ if it can have the triglyceride in mother's milk and make it into myelin.
10. The debate about breastfeeding and intelligence is over. BUT there are other important things to do over and above breastfeeding to enhance development.
11. Up to 6 months, milk is 7.4% fat, but at 12 months it is 10.7% (nearly 50% more). It might not be major for calorie requirement, but it is not used as fuel calories, it is used in the brain.

Reference List

(1) Gartner LM, Morton J, Lawrence RA, Naylor AJ, O'Hare D, Schanler RJ et al. Breastfeeding and the use of human milk. Pediatrics 2005 February;115(2):496-506.
(2) WHO. Systematic reviews: Evidence on the long-term effects of breastfeeding. WHO 2007.
(3) Picciano MF. Human milk: nutritional aspects of a dynamic food. Biol Neonate 1998;74(2):84-93.
(4) Xanthou M. Immune protection of human milk. Biol Neonate 1998;74(2):121-33.
(5) Emmett PM, Rogers IS. Properties of human milk and their relationship with maternal nutrition. Early Hum Dev 1997 October 29;49 Suppl:S7-S28.
(6) Schanler RJ. Suitability of human milk for the low-birthweight infant. Clinics in Perinatology 1995 March;22(1):207-22.
(7) Xu RJ. Development of the newborn GI tract and its relation to colostrum/milk intake: a review. Reprod Fertil Dev 1996;8(1):35-48.
(8) Habicht JP. Expert consultation on the optimal duration of exclusive breastfeeding: the process, recommendations, and challenges for the future. Adv Exp Med Biol 2004;554:79-87.:79-87.
(9) Caspi A, Williams B, Kim-Cohen J, Craig IW, Milne BJ, Pouldon R et al. Moderation of breastfeeding effects on the IQ by genetic variation in fatty acid metabolism. PNAS 2007;104(47):18860-5.
(10) Kramer MS, Aboud F, Mironova E, Vanilovich I, Platt RW, Matush L et al. Breastfeeding and child cognitive development: new evidence from a large randomized trial. Archives Of General Psychiatry 2008 May;65(5):578-84.
(11) Mandel D, Lubetzky R, Dollberg S, Barak S, Mimouni FB. Fat and Energy Contents of Expressed Human Breast Milk in Prolonged Lactation. Pediatrics 2005 September 1;116(3):e432-e435.

WAYS OF FEEDING PRETERM BABIES

Premie babies need breastmilk even more than full term babies!

Feeding you premie will depend on your own baby's needs, development and situation. It will also depend on your hospital's methods and policies.

Do insist on breastmilk as much as you possibly can!

Also, avoid bottle feeding if you possibly can !

For an extremely premature baby, there is a usual progression, and I shall explain these steps:

TPN ⟶ NGT/OGT ⟶ finger feed ⟶ cup feed ⟶ breastfeed

> **"TPN"** stands for Total Parenteral Nutrition, and means feeding your baby directly into the blood, through an intravenous line, bypassing the intestines. This is done when the gut is just too immature to be able to digest your milk. Though this is difficult and expensive, it is often necessary and life saving. Do start expressing your milk in the meantime! The colostrum is still safe to give.

My baby did not need   TPN   ....

My baby did need TPN: started   .... (date)

                            Ended   ....

                            Reason   ....

How to feed your premie breastmilk

In the previous chapter we looked at how to express milk. At 28 weeks of gestation your baby may struggle to latch onto the breast and may need your breastmilk through a tube into the stomach.

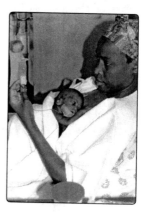

> A **nasogastric tube (NGT)** goes through the nose directly into the gut, and
>
> an **orogastric tube (OGT)** goes through the mouth straight to the stomach.
>
> There are reasons for both.

To get breastfeeding started, express two drops of milk for your premie to smell. Encourage her suckle on the breast at the same time as you have the tube in her nose or mouth.

OGT/NGT feeding

Cup-feeding: you may need to cup-feed, or feed your milk with a teaspoon (1). Avoid using a bottle as it is stressful for your baby. The nurses can <u>cup feed</u> or spoon feed your milk when you are not there.

If the baby is struggling to suck, a syringe can be put into the side of her mouth while she is on the breast.

To encourage sucking, you can try **"finger-feeding"** where a very fine tube is taped onto your finger, to teach her sucking skills. Alternatively, while the baby is sucking on a finger, small amounts of breastmilk can be fed into the side of her mouth with a syringe. If the baby cannot breastfeed yet, give her food via these methods while at the breast.

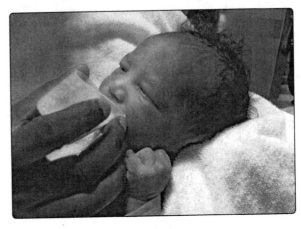

Cup feeding

What about bottle feeding?

Many hospitals use bottles to feed premies, it is convenient and one can know how much food the baby gets. But bottle-feeding is stressful for any baby as she cannot co-ordinate the muscles she uses for sucking and breathing: see diagram below, of oxygen saturations during bottle and breastfeeding (2),

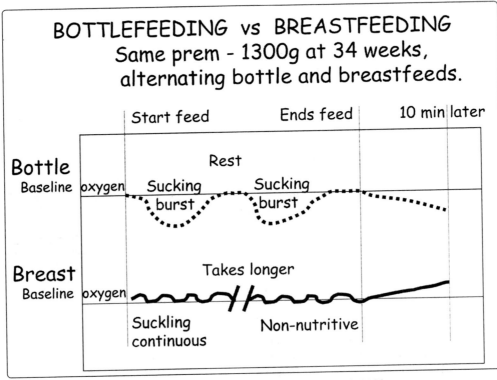

Adapted from Paula Meier, Nursing Fesearch 1988

Some of the muscles for sucking from a bottle are the same muscles used for breathing. (Try swallowing from a straw and breathing at the same time!) So your baby sucks from the bottle until she runs out of air, then she breathes and rests, then she sucks some more. A baby also gets too much milk, too fast from a bottle. This is not helpful to her (3).

<u>Important</u> – **suck and suckle are not the same.**

Babies can suckle from a breast and breathe at the same time!

In the past, it was believed that suckling from a breast was more tiring for the baby, and the bottle was recommended. Actually, bottle feeding is more stressful and breastfeeding uses less energy (4).

<u>What about pacifiers or "dummies"?</u>

Pacifiers are often used to calm a crying baby, which is helpful if you cannot be there. It is important that tiny babies do not cry so that their stress levels are not increased. Pacifiers are often used as a compromise (5;6). If mother and baby are kept together, babies should not need to cry!

Pacifiers also stimulate the vagus nerve, which helps the stomach empty faster. This may not be helpful as the baby's tummy should not empty too quickly (7). If the baby is in "separation distress" the gut may shut down due to somatostatin, and then this effect is very helpful.

Pacifiers are discouraged in international "Baby Friendly Hospitals", for good reasons. Like the nipple or teat of a bottle, the nipple of a pacifier is often too hard and too big for a premature baby. Bottles and pacifiers use a sucking method which uses cheek muscles instead of the jaw muscles used in breastfeeding. Sucking on a pacifier or bottle strengthens the wrong muscles and the baby cannot latch onto the nipple properly. The result may be that the mother gets cracked, sore nipples.

The cheek development is also not good for later speech development.

Pacifiers can also cause dental deformation, as the teeth can be pushed crookedly in the jaw. When a baby is sucking on a pacifier or bottle while lying flat, saliva collects in the back of the mouth. This fluid may run into the Eustachian tube, which can cause middle ear infections.

I know that the use of pacifiers is a sensitive issue! As parents you should be given the information on both the advantages and the disadvantages, and then be allowed to make your own choices.

<u>How much and how often to feed a FULLTERM baby?</u>

How babies are fed varies enormously from hospital to hospital. Let us first look at a full term baby, then at how your premie should feed.

The "daily amount required" for a baby to grow is about 2.5 fl oz of milk per lb of weight per day (150 - 160 ml per kg) . The average full-term newborn weighs about 6 or 7 lb, so let us use 16 fl oz as the daily amount required. When the baby comes home and is feeding three hourly, she needs 2 fl oz each time. The problem is that there is no research evidence to show that this is the size of the stomach. The research available suggests that the stomach size is only about 1/2 to 2/3 fl oz – that is only 2 tablespoons! (8–10) It means that the baby really needs to feed once every hour and take a smaller amount.

The stomach is elastic, and can stretch. It behaves a bit like a balloon; when you stretch it several times, it loses its ability to shrink back to the normal small size, and becomes bigger. Are we stretching our babies' stomachs too much? (Imagine your own discomfort after eating too big a meal.)

When the baby breastfeeds, she stimulates the breast with rapid mouth movements to produce a "milk ejection reflex". The volume of this is 1 fl oz at most, in all mothers, no matter how big or small their breasts are. Research has also shown that babies do not swallow the whole amount and the breast stores the remainder for later (11;12).

The "one hourly feeding schedule" also matches other biological behaviors. The stomach empties a milk meal in 60 minutes. Also, the normal sleep cycle of a baby is approximately 60 minutes. The sugar content (lactose) of milk lasts just 60 minutes. The proteins in milk come in very low concentration, so they also need topping up every hour.

As a mother, I can hear you say that feeding once every hour would be far too demanding. Actually, and surprisingly, it is much easier, quicker and saves time!

A "normal" breastfeeding session (meaning one dose every three hours) takes about 20 to 25 minutes. This is because the baby has to stimulate four or five ejection reflexes in succession to get the milk she knows she needs. Let us leave aside the burping time and the comfort time, and just say it takes 20 minutes each time. If you do that 8 times a day, you spend about 3 hours per day feeding your baby.

Now, the very first ejection reflex takes less than 2 minutes for the baby to produce (11;13), and the baby can swallow it in about half a minute, without problems. Quick and easy: two and a half minutes, 24 times a day, is just one hour you have spent feeding your baby. You have saved yourself two hours, and you do not need to burp her, because the stomach is relaxed and able to deal with the air by itself.

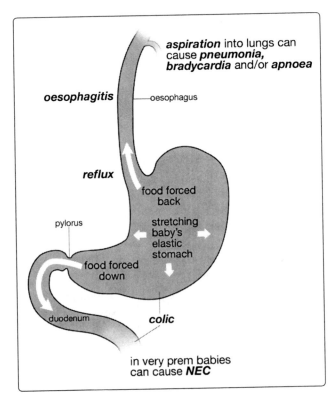

Problems caused by feeding baby too much.

How much and how often to feed your PRETERM baby?

Most hospitals start feeding extremely small babies once an hour, then every two hours and aim to send babies home feeding three hourly. Having understood why fullterm babies need small amounts often, how much more does this apply to premies?

Premies have very small stomachs, proportional to the physical size of the baby. "Reflux" is common in premature babies; this happens when stomach contents go back up the esophagus and cause burning pain (14). Apnea may also be caused this way. In many hospitals, babies are routinely treated for reflux, even operated on. Everyone knows babies burp, or "spit up" after a meal, and this has long been regarded as "normal". But is it necessary?

At the same time as excess milk comes back up as reflux, it goes right through the stomach into the small bowel, (duodenum) where it may also cause problems. This large volume may also be a cause of the colic that so many full-term babies experience.

The premie is less resilient and copes poorly with stress. Babies who are fed small amounts frequently have less colic.

> **A premie's stomach and body are more sensitive than those of a fullterm baby.**

As the stomach empties in 60 minutes, the blood sugar level also starts to fall. Hospitals often do routine heel prick tests on newborn and premature babies to check for low blood sugar. The heel prick is a stressful and painful event for the baby, and calories are used for crying. This may be one reason why small babies grow so slowly. When the blood sugar level is low, the baby is given sugar water or extra sugar in the drip. If your baby is "hypoglycemic", it could be translated as "hungry"! (She had 24 hour continuous feeding inside you!) If your baby gets frequent, small feeds, she may not need this extra sugar, nor the routine heel pricks.

Nurses are often busy; your baby needs you, her mom, to be there to feed her

> **There are good reasons to feed your premie once an hour.**

regularly. Possibly premies do not grow well because they are not fed small amounts often enough. Premies in Skin-to-Skin Contact often grow at the rate of 2/3 oz a day compared to 1/3 oz a day for a baby in an incubator. Feeding and holding your baby in Skin-to-Skin Contact will shorten your stay in hospital because your baby will grow faster.

FOR MOMS:

My baby had a feeding tube   started .... (date)

                                           ended ....

The tube was in the .... (nose, mouth)

I first finger fed my baby............................... (date) at .... days old.

I first cup-fed my baby .... (date) at .... days old.

I first BREASTFED my baby................................ (date) at .... days old.

My NICU policy was to feed at ....(2 hourly, 3hourly, 4 hourly)

My baby got feeds at.. intervals

(Describe baby's comfort level after feeds)

....

....

....

....

....

....

....

....

....

....

....

....

....

....

....

....

....

....

....

Fine Print Page – Feeding Your Preterm baby

1. This is a technical review, and covers cup-feeding evidence pages 4, and 62-64. It can be downloaded from internet: http://www.who.int/child_adolescent_health/documents/9241595094/en/index.html   and covers all aspects of feeding a low birth weight infant.
2. Babies were 32 weeks, and the same babies were studied bottle-feeding and breastfeeding. Bottle-feeding caused hypoxia.
3. Different muscles are used to suck from a bottle and suckle from a breast, despite a teat modified to resemble the breast nipple.
4. Quote "There were 2 episodes of apnea (breath pause more than 20 seconds) and 20 episodes of oxygen desaturation (PaO 2< 90%) during bottle-feeding and none during breastfeeding. We conclude that breastfeed-ing is a more physiological feeding method for the preterm infant and bottle-feeding may be more stressful."
5–7. There are benefits of pacifiers, but these have only been studied in the short term, not the long term. The effect on breastfeeding is however widely accepted, though hard to prove.
    NOTE: the recommendations on small frequent feedings originate from Nils Bergman's own observations and research synthesis. The following three publications are the only ones known to me, and they establish the small stomach size. I welcome articles and other research on this, and the opportunity to conduct clinical trials.
8. This paper describes the stomach growing as seen on ultrasound. It grows in proportion to the baby, and though a volume is not provided, the data can be used to calculate a volume of 12 mls before birth.
9. Very similar study, but shows full term fetus swallowing over 30 minutes to fill stomach to about 12 mls, and then gastric peristalsis emptying the stomach in about 5 – 10 minutes.
10. In this study, stillborn babies and those dying in the first week were studied, and the stomach stretched to full capacity with water pressure … volumes of about 15 – 20 mls. So unstretched it would be 12 ml !!!
11–12. This paper describes an ultrasound of a breast during feeding. The milk ejection reflex (MER) fills the ducts, and milk can be seen flowing out, but also back if not drunk by baby. The volume of the breast was meas-ured, and varied greatly, depending on how much of the reflex the baby swallowed at that feed. The weight gain of the baby shows also the volume of milk produced, and is 30 mls for the first MER, and then 20ml or so for each subsequent, the whole feed taking 15 minutes.
13. Here are many papers studying this, but this one shows nicely how very common reflux is. But it also shows the effects of feeding two hourly or three hourly or four hourly. Milk buffers acid, and so to get acid reflux, this only happens three hours after a milk meal. Babies that breastfed frequently may get reflux, but it is not acid reflux!!

Reference List

(1) Edmond KT, Bahl R. Optimal feeding of low-birth-weight infants technical review. WHO 2006;1-131.
(2) Meier P. Bottle- and breast-feeding: effects on transcutaneous oxygen pressure and temperature in preterm infants. Nursing Research 1988 January;37(1):36-41.
(3) Mizuno K, Fujimaki K, Sawada M. Sucking behavior at breast during the early newborn period affects later breast-feeding rate and duration of breast-feeding. Pediatrics International: Official Journal Of The Japan Pediatric Society 2004 February;46(1):15-20.
(4) Chen CH, Wang TM, Chang HM, Chi CS. The effect of breast - and bottle-feeding on oxygen saturation and body temperature in preterm infants. J Hum Lact 2000 February;16(1):21-7.
(5) Anderson GC. [Skin-to-skin: the kangaroo technic in western Europe]. Servir 1989 November;37(6):316-20.
(6) Pinelli J, Symington A. How rewarding can a pacifier be? A systematic review of nonnutritive sucking in preterm infants. Neonatal Netw 2000 December;19(8):41-8.
(7) Widstrom AM, Marchini G, Matthiesen AS, Werner S, Winberg J, Uvnas-Moberg K. Nonnutritive sucking in tube-fed preterm infants: effects on gastric motility and gastric contents of somatostatin. J Pediatr Gastroen-terol Nutr 1988 July;7(4):517-23.
(8) Goldstein I, Reece EA, Yarkoni S, Wan M, Green JL, Hobbins JC. Growth of the fetal stomach in normal pregnancies. Obstet Gynecol 1987 October;70(4):641-4.
(9) Naveed M, Manjunath CS, Sreenivas, V. An autopsy Study of Relationship between Perinatal Stomach Ca-pacity and Birth Weight. Indian J Gastroenterol 1992;11(4):156-8.
(10) Sase M, Miwa I, Sumie M, Nakata M, Sugino N, Okada K et al. Gastric emptying cycles in the human fetus. American Journal Of Obstetrics And Gynecology 2005 September;193(3 Pt 2):1000-4.
(11) Prime DK, Geddes DT, Hartmann PE. Oxytocin: Milk ejection and maternal-infant well-being. Hale & Hartmann's Textbook of Human Lactation 2007;141-55.
(12) Ramsay DT, Kent JC, Owens RA, Hartmann PE. Ultrasound Imaging of Milk Ejection in the Breast of Lac-tating Women. Pediatrics 2004 February;113(2):361-7.
(13) Lopez-Alonso M, Moya MJ, Cabo JA, Ribas J, M, Silny J et al. Twenty-four-hour esophageal impedance-pH monitoring in healthy preterm neonates: rate and characteristics of acid, weakly acidic, and weakly alkaline gastroesophageal reflux. Pediatrics 2006 August;118(2):e299-e308.
(14) Lopez-Alonso M, Moya MJ, Cabo JA, Ribas J, M, Silny J et al. Twenty-four-hour esophageal impedance-pH monitoring in healthy preterm neonates: rate and characteristics of acid, weakly acidic, and weakly alkaline gastroesophageal reflux. Pediatrics 2006 August;118(2):e299-e308.

BREASTFEEDING YOUR PRETERM BABY

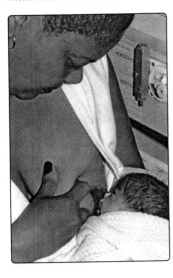 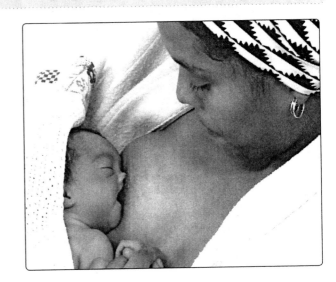

The huge benefits from exclusively breastfeeding from birth to six months are well-researched and proven (1;2). In the first section we looked at the benefits from the actual breastmilk. The food is only a small part of what your baby is getting from you to help her grow.

The physical action of breastfeeding itself produces benefits and helps brain growth. Each of the sensations that the baby receives in Skin-to-Skin Contact together with the breastmilk produces different types of intelligence.

Being in the right place on mom's chest and breastfeeding makes the brain grow best as the baby feels SAFE and LOVED (see page 81, the diagram "Sensations that Wire the Brain"). By breastfeeding, you are wiring your baby's brain for health and intelligence for her whole life.

Can tiny premies breastfeed?

Yes, they can!

This may seem surprising, but if we look at the capabilities of the premature baby, we see that premies are not as helpless as many believe.

From 28 weeks gestation onwards a premie can suckle on the breast (3-5).

If your baby is born prematurely, you need to have some idea of what she can do. Each baby is unique, so there will be variation according to how premature your baby was born.

Here is the basic biology of what your baby would be doing if she were still in your womb.

> By 18 – 24 weeks the baby inside her mom is able to swallow amniotic fluid.
>
> By 22 weeks she can pout her lips (so as to close her lips to get a seal when suckling).
>
> By full term a baby has practiced all the breastfeeding behaviors for many weeks, and is ready to breastfeed.

When a baby is born prematurely, these behaviors are present but not well practiced. The premie develops skills in the following order (exact age individually variable) (5).

> By 28 weeks gestation she has a strong rooting reflex and is able to suck, swallow and breathe, but only briefly and these may not be co-ordinated.
>
> By 31 weeks, there is repeated swallowing of milk from the breast.
>
> By 30–32 weeks the baby can co-ordinate sucking, swallowing and breathing.
>
> By 34 weeks the baby can breastfeed fully (but some much earlier!).

Your baby has a strong gag reflex to protect her from getting milk down her airway (6). If she has been suctioned at birth or had a feeding tube, she may gag if anything, even the breast, is placed in her mouth (7;8). Go slowly and gently.

Keep your baby in the right <u>place</u> (in Skin-to-Skin Contact) and she will show the right <u>behaviors</u>. These are called "rooting behaviors" or just "cues".

Pre-feeding cues

> licking her lips, mouth movements;
>
> turning her head and looking towards your breast;
>
> smelling your nipple, touching it with her hands;
>
> moving hand to mouth, nuzzling mouth to breast.

Keep your baby close to the nipple, and she may start to breastfeed all by herself!

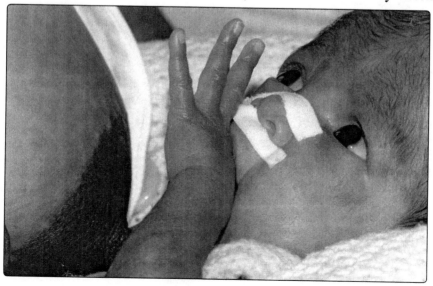

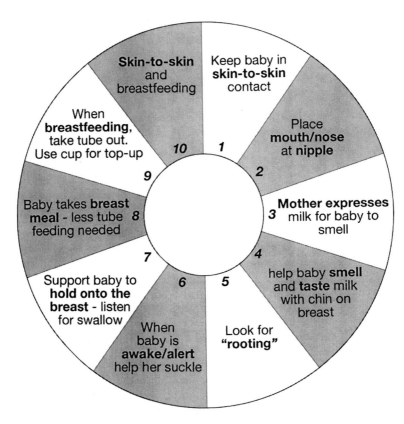

This wheel (adapted from Persson) describes the ten small steps to breast-feeding (9;10):

1 Baby must be in Skin-to-Skin Contact, close to breast.

2 Baby smells the nipple.

3 Baby smells the breastmilk.

4 Baby tastes the breastmilk on the nipple.

5 Baby will make mouth movements called rooting (premies may only sip the milk at first).

6 Baby must be awake and alert for suckling.

7 Baby latches on and swallows milk.

8 First breastmilk meal. Steps 1–7 go fast for full term babies, premies may need successive alert times with sleep cycling between each.

9 Baby feeds frequently, (for premies every 60–90 minutes).

10 Mom and baby are together continuously.

Mom, be encouraged if your baby is doing <u>any</u> of these tiny steps. Maybe you could write a date and time next to each one so that you can see her progress. Dad, you can be a wonderful help to your wife by encouraging her with breastfeeding. The progress may seem very slow and frustrating for her.

Mom, here are some ways to encourage breastfeeding.

- With fingers, gently rub in small circles near the outside of your baby's mouth, and on cheek area near jaw line
- Using smallest finger, gently rub same areas *inside* mouth
- Massage soft tissue under chin bone to stimulate muscles used for breastfeeding
- Encourage baby to suck her fist
- As often as baby is awake, keep her at your breasts.

Again, you may need to call in a lactation consultant or breastfeeding support person to help you to get your premie latching and breastfeeding properly. It may take time. There are MANY excellent books on breastfeeding so I will not go into more detail here (11).

As the baby suckles, the nipple is pulled deep into her mouth. The action of suckling stimulates the back of the mouth, the soft palate and soothes the baby as it aids the release of oxytocin. Because she is soothed and calmed, her gut will absorb all her food. You need to hold your baby "tummy to mommy" and she needs a good amount of your areola inside her mouth for a proper latch. Try to relax and this will help your baby to relax as well. Listen for her swallowing to know that she is drinking properly.

Always put the baby next to your breast to smell the nipple and taste the milk even if

> **The more often your baby feeds, the more milk is produced, so feed her small amounts often.**

it is only a drop. All newborns, even tiny premies, have a strong sense of smell. You want your baby to smell and taste the right and expected food, breast milk and link it to you, her mom. Her small hands make kneading movements on your breasts, and her tiny attempts at suckling, will help towards your breasts producing her next meal.

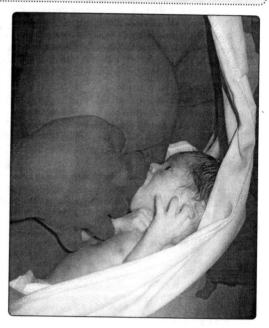

Fine Print Page – Breastfeeding Your Preterm

1. This statement is not generally believed … but the evidence has been building up over the years, and it is only recently that there is enough of it for the World Health Organisation to "put its head on the block" ! From abstract: "WHO (to) change … to a recommendation to promote exclusive breastfeeding for six months.". Further "The amount of scientific evidence available was more than is often available for policy decisions in health, but much less than desirable to address issues of generalizability across and within populations."

2. A Cochrane review allows only the strictest possible evidence criteria, and is therefore worded very cau-tiously. This paper chose only 20 best studies from 2688 articles, and ends by saying that bigger and better studies are needed to "confirm the health benefits reported thus far, and to investigate other potential effects on health and development, especially over the long term."

3–5. These papers introduce the work of Kerstin Hedberg-Nyqvist. Conclusion from Ref 5; "Very preterm infants have the capacity for early development of oral motor competence that it sufficient for establishment of full breastfeeding at a low postmenstrual age."

6. Authors define breastfeeding as the "physiological norm", during which "swallowing occurred nonrandomly between breaths and did not interfere with breathing."

7–8. This is a review of routines, quote: "Many common care practices during labor, birth, and the immediate post-partum period impact the fetal to neonatal transition, including … suctioning protocols". And it summa-rizes by "routine suctioning of infants at birth has not been found to be beneficial." Widstrom writes that the sequence of prefeeding behavior described in the Skin-to-Skin Contact chapter "was disrupted in children who had undergone gastric suction."

9–10. Wahlberg first published "Persson's Wheel", more accessible version with the science explained is in Meier's chapter.

11. Biological Nurturing expands some of these concepts: http://www.biologicalnurturing.com/

Reference List

(1) Habicht JP. Expert consultation on the optimal duration of exclusive breastfeeding: the process, recommenda-tions, and challenges for the future. Adv Exp Med Biol 2004;554:79-87.:79-87.

(2) Kramer MS, Kakuma R. The optimal duration of exclusive breastfeeding: a systematic review. Adv Exp Med Biol 2004;554:63-77.:63-77.

(3) Nyqvist KH, Rubertsson C, Ewald U, Sjoden P. Development of the Preterm Infant Breastfeeding Behavior Scale (PIBBS): a study of nurse-mother agreement. J HUM LACT 1996 September;12(3):207-19.

(4) Nyqvist KH, Sj+¦d+n PO, Ewald U. The development of preterm infants' breastfeeding behavior. Early Human Development 1999 July;55(3):247-64.

(5) Nyqvist KH. Early attainment of breastfeeding competence in very preterm infants. Acta Paediatrica 2008 June;97(6):776-81.

(6) Goldfield EC, Richardson MJ, Lee KG, Margetts S. Coordination of sucking, swallowing, and breathing and oxy-gen saturation during early infant breast-feeding and bottle-feeding. Pediatr Res 2006 October 28;60(4):450-5.

(7) Mercer JS, Erickson-Owens DA, Graves B, Haley MM. Evidence-based practices for the fetal to newborn transi-tion. Journal of Midwifery and Womens Health 2007;52(3):262-72.

(8) Widstrom AM, Ransjo-Arvidson AB, Christensson K, Matthiesen AS, Winberg J, Uvnas-Moberg K. Gastric suc-tion in healthy newborn infants. Effects on circulation and developing feeding behaviour. Acta Paediatr Scand 1987 July;76(4):566-72.

(9) Meier PP, Mangurten HH. Breastfeeding the Pre-Term Infant. In: Riordan JM, Auerbach KG, editors. Breast-feeding and Human Lactation.Boston: Jones & Bartlett; 1993. p. 253-78.

(10) Wahlberg V. The "Kangaroo method" and breastfeedng in low birth weight babies. Nytt on U-landshalsovard 1991;5(3):22-7.

(11) Colson S. Biological nurturing. Biological Nurturing 2005

HOW THE BRAIN DEVELOPS AND WORKS: NEUROSCIENCE

The brain is the most important part of your baby!

It will make her what she will become.

Early experience makes the brain what it is.

Your baby's brain is wired by you!

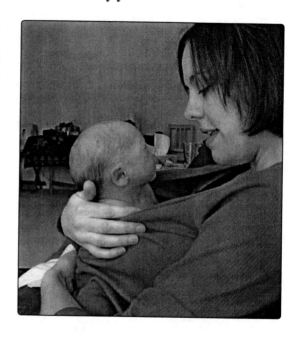

The brain is a sensory organ; it collects signals which fire sensitive cells called neurons. As they fire, they wire connections and circuits in the brain.

By 28 weeks the fetus has the most nerve cells she will ever have. The neurons will move and be coated in myelin to speed up the sending of messages in the brain. She will keep the neurons and circuits that fire often and lose those that do not fire.

These circuits need sleep to organize properly.

They develop in layers, that make a baby develop physically, emotionally, intellectually and socially at the same time.

In her mother's womb, the baby is already collecting messages or "sensations" of touch, sound, and warmth from her mother. When she is born she is expecting these familiar sounds.

What a shock then to be separated from her mother, and so the baby feels unsafe, and her brain fires and wires for stress and avoidance. Premature babies are even more sensitive and struggle even more to find their balance so they need Skin-to-Skin Contact even more than full term babies. A baby that was separated from Mom for a long time at birth may struggle to connect with people later. This poorer social development has long-term effects on health.

We need to do all that we can to protect the premie's brain from harm. We also need to positively help her brain growth to be healthy.

Being a caring parent is a vital and wonderful "job" for the next few years.

Your baby needs you to do it!

Note: This chapter may seem complicated, but there are practical things that you can do to help your baby's brain development.

To understand your baby's needs it may be helpful to know how her brain has been growing, and why protecting the brain is so important for the <u>quality</u> of her survival.

How the brain grows and develops from conception:

In the first days after conception a tube forms with a swelling at one end which is the beginning of the brain and the spinal cord. In the tube there are neurons (or nerve cells) which collect information and conduct messages. The neurons are tree-shaped, and both branches and roots make a network in the brain, with connections to the body. Some nerves are covered with myelin, a fatty membrane, which speeds up the sending of messages. To make myelin requires special fatty acids found in human breastmilk.

<u>Inside mother, during pregnancy</u>

From 0–14 weeks the genes mostly decide your baby's development. After that, experience and sensations are more important in deciding how the brain grows.

Between 10 to 14 weeks the brain appears and the eyes start to develop.

By 20 weeks all brain structures are in place and working!

By 23 weeks the fetus is conscious and aware. Her tiny ears hear and her eyes react to light. She can taste, swallow, and suck her thumb to soothe herself.

By 28 weeks the fetus has the most nerve cells she will ever have. No more are produced after this (except in two small areas). These cells still need to move to their final positions and to branch and connect to other nerve cells. By 28 weeks the brain is developed well enough for the baby to survive outside the womb – on her mother. (The lungs and other organs may need help.)

During the last third of pregnancy development is about connecting the neurons (1).

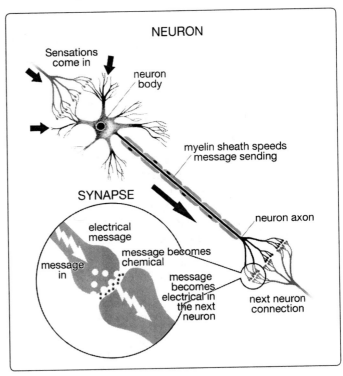

> **"Cells that fire together, wire together,
> and those that don't, won't." – Carla Shatz**

Those nerve cells that are not fired-wired, are removed, they are unnecessary and in the way! And so 50% of the nerve cells that the baby had at 28 weeks have disappeared by 40 weeks (2).

> **"Use it or lose it"**

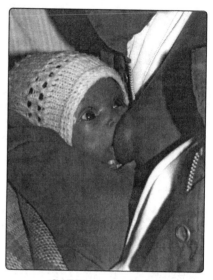

The nerve cells in your baby's brain are <u>expecting</u> certain messages at particular times during development. Your baby is expecting the sound of your voice and heart beat, your smell, and the sight of your face. These will make her feel safe, and protected. She is expecting quiet muffled sounds in her ears and darkness for her developing eyes. These expectations are linked to basic pathways on which later pathways will be built.

In Skin-to-Skin Contact the baby feels SAFE.

The mother's body helps the baby's body to find a physically healthy balance or stability. This sets healthy set points for her heart rate, blood pressure and oxygen saturation. If the baby is later stressed, she will be able to cope better and return to stability or "self-regulate".

'SAFE' on mom's chest

The same thing happens with the baby's emotional balance. New neuroscience has shown that the baby's brain translates all sensations into emotions. These help the baby to know which people or situations are good. Emotion is core to making any decision. Good is felt as reward which the baby seeks or approaches. Feeling SAFE fires the basic brain pathway to approach (3;4) so the baby will open her eyes, even at a very early gestational age and make eye-to-eye contact with her mother to bond and attach to her. Your baby is conscious and aware and is an emotional being with needs just like yours. Your emotions shape your baby's emotions (7).

When did your baby first open her eyes?

A baby separated from her mother will feel UNSAFE.

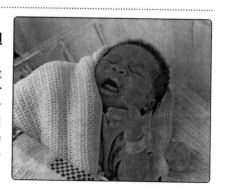

She will cry, her blood pressure and heart rate will increase and she will struggle with her breathing. She will not have help to set healthy physical set points. On an emotional level separation fires the avoidance pathway in the brain. This baby will look inwards and struggle to cope emotionally, and will avoid eye contact.

Repeating these patterns wires the circuits of the baby's early personality. The ability to decide appropriately to approach or avoid is the foundation for her health and well-being now, and her mental health later (5;6).

Your baby's brain is wired by you!

You, Mom and Dad, need to make sure that your baby's brain is wired for good things, not bad.

**Being caring parents is a vital and wonderful "job" for the next few years.
Your baby needs you to do it!**

If your baby is born early, these needs for gentle and peaceful safe sensations may not be met. For a premie, brain development may now be in the busy, noisy NICU, in an incubator, separated from mother. No wonder being born prematurely is such a shock for her! The messages the brain receives are unexpected and frightening. The baby will withdraw, and therefore fire avoidance pathways in the brain.

**So how can you help your baby's brain to develop properly?
Give your baby Skin-to-Skin Contact**

It is Skin-to-Skin Contact which is the expected and therefore most important sensation after birth. Almost all the healthy sensations are provided on mom's chest. Skin-to-skin contact also stimulates the baby to breastfeed (8). This way all the good sensations are provided!
The baby's brain collects all the sensations together and organizes them to make sense of her world and wires her brain for health and well-being and calmness.

This skin-to-skin holding and breastfeeding is what is feeding your baby's brain.

"The brain is designed to be sculpted into its final configuration by the effects of early experiences." – *Martin Teicher* **(14)**

Which of these facts were new to you?

....

....

....

....

....

Sleep is very important for brain wiring, state organization and memory formation, as we shall see in the next chapter.

SENSATIONS THAT WIRE BRAIN

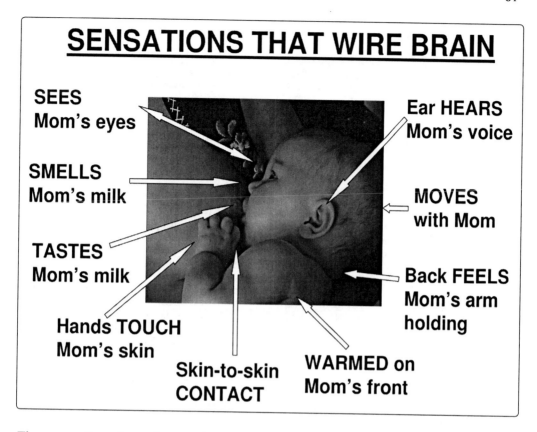

SEES
Mom's eyes

SMELLS
Mom's milk

TASTES
Mom's milk

Hands TOUCH
Mom's skin

Skin-to-skin CONTACT

Ear HEARS
Mom's voice

MOVES
with Mom

Back FEELS
Mom's arm
holding

WARMED on
Mom's front

These sensations depend on a primary caregiver, usually the mother.

Eye-to-eye contact with her mother sparks the part of the brain (the amygdala), which helps the baby bond with her mom and grow her emotional intelligence. Face-to-face contact sparks the brain pathways for belonging and social attachment.

Smell is probably the strongest sense in tiny babies. She smells your breast and breastmilk which are familiar and calming. The smell of breastmilk sends messages to the stomach to release enzymes to digest the milk (9;10).

She tastes your milk – exactly what she needs to grow.

Her hands feel the softness of your skin. Often a mother will hold her baby's tiny hand. Messages reach the mothers brain, to release the hormone oxytocin. This is the love hormone, but it also releases milk and calms mother (11;12).

The baby's skin feels the mothers' skin, and this sends messages to the front of the baby's brain (the frontal lobe cortex) to say that she is safe and can relax. This wires her amygdala or emotional brain for health and "approach" behavior (4).

Skin-to-Skin Contact makes baby feel warm and so she feels safe (13).

Your arm around her back holding and containing her stimulates the part of her brain for deep touch, making her feel that she belongs and that she is loved and safe.

Mom and baby move together, and this is familiar and reassuring.

Her ears hear your voice and heartbeat – so familiar and soothing from all her months inside you.

Fine Print Page – How the Brain Develops

1. Carla Shatz studied how vision developed in fetal kittens, she blocked the firing of the neurons, and the kit-tens were born with perfect eyes, but they were blind.
2. This human study shows the higher number of neurons babies have compared to adults, albeit in a specific area of the brain.
3–5. Amodio describes the BAS (Behavioral Approach System) in detail. The two articles by Schore are an exten-sive review of this neuroscience, and pages 25 – 33 in "secure attachment" deal with the skin contact and tac-tile effects on brain pathways, and the subsequent regulation and orientation behavior.
6. Panksepp's research bridges basic brain neuroscience with psychology and psychiatry, and this book is a de-tailed treatise of this work in mammals. He says "use it or lose it" (page 17), but also summarizes developmen-tal trajectories, contrasting effects of "social comfort" against "separation distress" (page 263).
7. The first half of this book describes how the mother baby interactions and the positive sensory environment shape the baby's brain, its intelligence, and its ability to communicate and speak.
8. In this study, authors show that "Early postpartum mother-baby Skin-to-Skin Contact had a powerful influ-ence (P<0.001) over the duration of exclusive breastfeeding up to 4-6 months and was found to be more sig-nificant than early initiation of breastfeeding (P<0.05)." This reflects early influences on brain pathways that make breast-feeding easier. Smell is especially important … as follows:
9–10. Porter has studied olfaction (smell) in the newborn period, and shows how important this is for the newborn. This is important, because we adults have lost the olfactory capacity babies have, and so ignore it. But babies depend on it !!! The sense of security the baby has comes in part from the continuity provided by smells in the uterus (amniotic fluid) to the Skin-to-Skin Contact and then the breasts (milk).
11–12. Kerstin Uvnas-Moberg describes the "love hormone" oxytocin, the book reference (11) is written for a lay reader. 'It seems that tactile, olfactory, visual, and perhaps other types of sensory stimuli contribute to the adaptive changes in both mother and infant. Central oxytocinergic mechanisms activated in connection with birth and breastfeeding seem to be involved in the behavioral changes".
13. This is the introductory article of a hard cover journal, all of which deals with the sensory environment. Quote: "Future NICU design should recognize that the baby must spend most of its time in its mother's arms to get the full benefit of her sensory environment as experienced throughout our evolution."
14. This article refers to the normal brain development described briefly in this chapter, but goes on to describe mala-daptive changes that follow from stress and trauma.

Reference List

(1) Shatz CJ. The developing brain. Sci Am 1992 September;267(3):60-7.
(2) Abitz M, Nielsen RD, Jones EG, Laursen H, Graem N, Pakkenberg B. Excess of neurons in the human new-born mediodorsal thalamus compared with that of the adult. Cerebral Cortex (New York, N Y : 1991) 2007 November 11;17(11):2573-8.
(3) Amodio DM, Master SL, Yee CM, Taylor SE. Neurocognitive components of the behavioral inhibition and acti-vation systems: Implications for theories of self-regulation. Psychophysiology 2008;45:11-1.
(4) Schore AN. Effects of a secure attachment relationship on right brain development, affect regulation, and infant mental health. Infant Mental Health Journal 2001;22(1-2):7-66.
(5) Schore AN. The effects of early relational trauma on right brain development, affect regulation, and infant mental health. Infant Mental Health Journal 2001;22(1-2):201-69.
(6) Panksepp J. Affective neuroscience. Oxford Univarsity Press; 1998.
(7) Greenspan SI, Shanker SG, Phil D. The First Idea: How symbols, language, and intelligence evolved from our primate ancestors to modern humans. 1st ed. Cambridge: Da Capo Press; 2006.
(8) Vaidya K, Sharma A, Dhungel S. Effect of early mother-baby close contact over the duration of exclusive breast-feeding. Nepal Medical College Journal: NMCJ 2005 December;7(2):138-40.
(9) Porter RH, Winberg J. Unique salience of maternal breast odors for newborn infants. Neurosci Biobehav Rev 1999;23(3):439-49.
(10) Porter RH. The biological significance of Skin-to-Skin Contact and maternal odours. Acta Paediatrica 2004 De-cember;93(12):1560-2.
(11) Uvnas-Moberg K, Francis R. The oxytocin factor: tapping the hormome of calm, love, and healing. MA Da Capo Press 2003;(Chapter 8 Nursing):93-103.
(12) Uvnas-Moberg K. Neuroendocrinology of the mother-child interaction. Trends In Endocrinology And Me-tabo-lism: TEM 1996 May;7(4):126-31.
(13) White RD. Mothers' arms--the past and future locus of neonatal care? Clin Perinatol 2004 June;31(2):383-7, ix.
(14) Teicher MH, Andersen SL, Polcari A, Anderson CM, Navalta CP. Developmental neurobiology of childhood stress and trauma. Psychiatr Clin North Am 2002 June;25(2):397-426.

PROTECT SLEEP

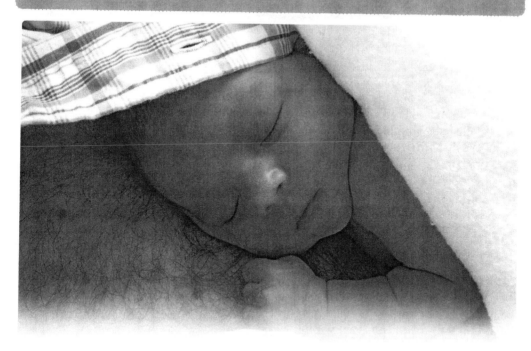

All babies need to sleep a lot.

Preterm babies need to sleep even more.

A premie in an incubator does not sleep properly.

A baby in Skin-to-Skin Contact will sleep better as she feels SAFE.

On your chest she will have the right temperature, and be hearing your heart beat, her head will be covered to shut out bright lights and to muffle sound. Her brain will have the chance to organize and form healthy pathways.

Babies' brains need sleep for memory formation and completing brain circuits.

Babies need to sleep and wake in cycles to get the best brain wiring. Good sleep cycling only happens when a baby is with her mother.

When a baby is sleeping she can use all her food energy for growing.

Do NOT wake her from quiet sleep.

Protect your baby's sleep and you will help her brain development.

Let us look at <u>what is happening inside the mother</u>. Before baby is born she sleeps a lot. In your womb, your baby has touch and contact, gentle movement and muffled sounds; your baby's brain collects these gentle messages and stores them. She follows her mother's day-night rhythm, but she also has her own sleep – wake cycles. Babies have two kinds of sleep states, even before birth.

The first is called "rapid-eye-movement sleep", or REM sleep. The baby is actually asleep, but the brain is very active and the eyes move under the eyelids. In her mother's womb, the baby's brain is firing to start making organized pathways (1;2). This happens without stimulations from the outside that normally make nerve cells fire. Inside the mother the baby's brain is not over-stimulated. The brain has time to organize all of the pathways that are being fired (3).

After REM or active sleep, the baby needs a time of quiet sleep. This is called "non-REM 4" (or NR4 in diagram). It can be recognized by a regular heart beat and breathing rate. During this time the brain pathways are completed and secured (4). After that, her brain is ready for another set of messages.

> **All babies need to sleep cycle to organize the wiring of their brains.**

Another period of REM sleep follows. If the baby is going to wake, it will usually be just before or during REM sleep. The cycling of REM and non-REM sleep is very important for growth and brain wiring.

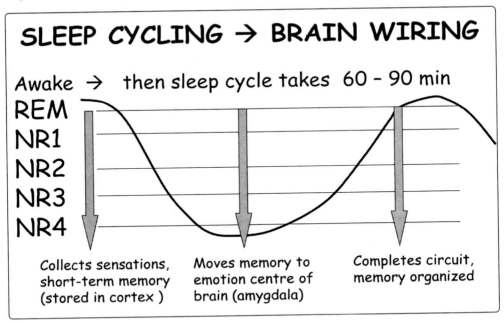

As the <u>premie is born too early</u>, she may be placed in a NICU with bright lights, lots of noise, distractions and many people. This is an overload of messages. The premie in an incubator does not sleep-cycle properly, and so cannot sort out all these messages. Because her sleep is disturbed, her memory formation and brain wiring are disorganized. She is alone and separated from her mother so she often cries until she is exhausted. When she eventually does sleep, she may sink into a very deep sleep, where she is so

SLEEP CYCLING
Separation vs Skin-to-Skin

Incubator   **SSC**

Chaotic behaviour pattern, little sleep | Regular sleep cycling

tired that she can even forget to breathe (apnea).

To help your premie sleep and brain wire properly, return her as closely as possible to the womb environment, or what she had inside you (5). Holding your baby in Skin-to-Skin Contact on your chest will help her to feel peaceful, and have sleep and wake cycling to control her state properly and so help healthy brain development (6;7).

At 27–30 weeks the premie baby is only alert for very short times. When the baby is awake, or in REM sleep, she is collecting messages which go to the surface of the brain (cortex). When she goes into quiet sleep (non-REM) the information is sent to the emotional centre of the brain (called the amygdala). Every physical sensation is stored with an emotion in the brain. When the baby starts to wake up, early REM sleep sends these messages to the front of the brain, which makes the decision to approach or avoid. This organized circuit of pathways is like a drawer system in which the memory is stored (8).

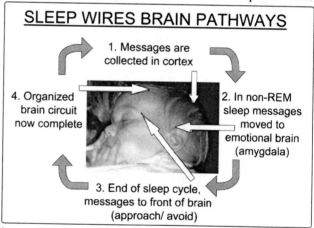

SLEEP WIRES BRAIN PATHWAYS

1. Messages are collected in cortex

2. In non-REM sleep messages moved to emotional brain (amygdala)

3. End of sleep cycle, messages to front of brain (approach/ avoid)

4. Organized brain circuit now complete

It is possible for you to learn how to tell which state your baby is in. When she is awake, her eyes are open and she is moving her arms and legs. She will then become drowsy and slow down. There may be small twitches of her fingers and face muscles. The distinctive "rapid eye movement" is not always easy to see. Her breathing and heart rate may be a bit irregular. Watch your baby for the small signs that tell you what state she is in, so that you know what the best care at that time will be.

**When she is in quiet sleep, her breathing is very even,
and her body is very still and calm.**

In quiet sleep she has a normal heart rate and her temperature tends to be more even than when she is awake. It is important not to disturb her at this time as she is sleeping quietly and is in an "organized" or unstressed state.

What a baby does and how she reacts depends on her state of being asleep or awake. The ability to control awake and asleep is called "state organization". One of the main problems for a premie separated from her mother is that she has poor state organization. This may contribute to premies having attention or concentration problems. In the diagram you can see how incubator babies swing chaotically from one extreme to the other. Crying is stressful and wastes calories; there is also a risk of bleeding in the brain. In deep sleep there is a risk of apnea. In Skin-to-Skin Contact, the mother's body settles and calms the baby. Your baby's state should cycle from good quality sleep to waking and feeding.

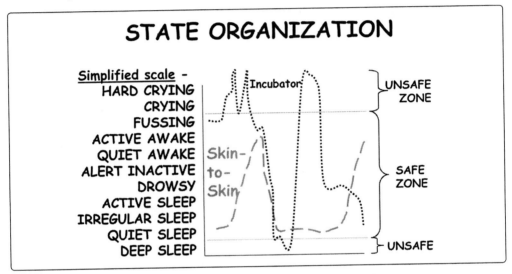

STATE ORGANIZATION

Simplified scale –
HARD CRYING
CRYING
FUSSING
ACTIVE AWAKE
QUIET AWAKE
ALERT INACTIVE
DROWSY
ACTIVE SLEEP
IRREGULAR SLEEP
QUIET SLEEP
DEEP SLEEP

Incubator
Skin-to-Skin
UNSAFE ZONE
SAFE ZONE
UNSAFE

Remember, good sleep cycling is vital for brain wiring and this only happens with mother. For the premie, quiet sleep is even more essential, as the brain is more sensitive.
Mom and baby also get into a rhythm of sleeping at the same time called ("sleep synchrony") (9).
The mom and baby act as "co-regulators" (10).

Your baby can be woken after REM sleep, but NOT during quiet sleep.
Protect your baby's sleep and you will help her brain development.

Premies sleep a lot and may need to be woken for feeding after a quiet sleep period. Small feeds every 60–90 minutes are better as they match the sleep cycle. Hold your baby in Skin-to-Skin Contact on your chest at least a full hour after a feed so that she can complete a full sleep-wake cycle, as well as absorb all of her food properly.

Fine Print Page – Protect Sleep

1–2.   These are both rather complex papers, but describe in detail what REM is and what it does. There is some controversy as always, but the need for REM and NREM sleep is undisputed.

3.   This article summarizes sleep development more practically, and covers most of the content of this chapter. Quote: "REM and NREM sleep cycling are essential for early neurosensory development, learning and mem-ory, and preservation of brain plasticity for the life of the individual."

4.   Sleep has been studied extensively, but there are fewer studies looking at the effect of Skin-to-Skin Contact on sleep. This paper concludes "The patterns demonstrated by the SSC group are analogous to more mature sleep organization. SSC may be used as an intervention to improve sleep organization in this population of preterm infants.".

5.   This study looked specifically at premature infants, confirming " ... a significant increase in sleep time for the neonates during Skin-to-skin Contact (with) less agitation, apnea, and bradycardia episodes and main-tained stable oxygen saturation ... safe even for very small neonates and is well tolerated".

6.   Feldman has published a number of follow-up studies, and in this shows that after SSC, premies at birth have "more mature state distribution and more organized sleep-wake cyclicity".

7.   This paper explains state organization, and also shows that fullterm babies sleep better when in Skin-to-Skin Contact

8.   Another complex paper... but describes in great detail how sleep cycling works... the hippocampus is studied here, and is closely linked to the amygdala.

9.   Sleep synchrony is also part of the contentious "co-sleeping debate"! It is safer for mother and baby to sleep together, but co-sleeping must also be done in a safe manner. (http://www.nd.edu/~jmckenn1/lab/faq.html)

10.   In animal studies, "mutual care giving between newborn and mothers" is described; Gene Cranston Anderson was perhaps the first to describe this in humans!

Reference List

(1)   Marks GA, Shaffery JP, Oksenberg A, Speciale SG, Roffwarg HP. A functional role for REM sleep in brain maturation. Behavioural Brain Research 1995 July;69(1-2):1-11.

(2)   Mirmiran M. The function of fetal/neonatal rapid eye movement sleep. Behavioural Brain Research 1995 July;69(1-2):13-22.

(3)   Graven S. Sleep and Brain Development. Clinics in Perinatology 2006;33:693-706.

(4)   Ludington-Hoe SM, Johnson MW, Morgan K, Lewis T, Gutman J, Wilson PD et al. Neurophysiologic Assessment of Neonatal Sleep Organization: Preliminary Results of a Randomized, Controlled Trial of Skin Contact With Preterm Infants. Journal of the American Academy of Child & Adolescent Psychiatry 2006 December;45(12):1455.

(5)   Messmer PR, Rodriguez S, Adams J, Wells-Gentry J, Washburn K, Zabaleta I et al. Effect of kangaroo care on sleep time for neonates. Pediatr Nurs 1997 July;23(4):408-14.

(6)   Feldman R, Weller A, Sirota L, Eidelman AI. Skin-to-Skin Contact (Kangaroo care) promotes self-regulation in premature infants: sleep-wake cyclicity, arousal modulation, and sustained exploration. Dev Psychol 2002 March;38(2):194-207.

(7)   Ferber SG, Makhoul IR. The effect of Skin-to-Skin Contact (kangaroo care) shortly after birth on the neuro-behavioral responses of the term newborn: a randomized, controlled trial. Pediatrics 2004 April;113(4):858-65.

(8)   Ji D, Wilson MA. Coordinated memory replay in the visual cortex and hippocampus during sleep. Nature Neuroscience 2007;10(1):100-7.

(9)   McKenna JJ, Mosko SS. Sleep and arousal, synchrony and independence, among mothers and infants sleeping apart and together (same bed): an experiment in evolutionary medicine. Acta Paediatr Suppl 1994 June;397:94-102.

(10)   Anderson GC. Risk in mother-infant separation postbirth. Image: Journal of Nursing Scholarship 1989;21(4):196-9.

SEPARATION AND STRESS

Being separated from mother is stressful for all babies.

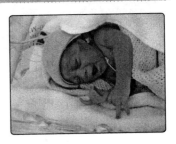

Your baby's security, her SAFE place is you, her mother. She will protest by crying if she is separated from you.

When a baby cries her heart rate and blood pressure go up, and oxygen saturation goes down.

If a preterm baby cries she is at increased risk for a brain bleed.

If she cries for too long your baby may go into despair behavior.

When babies are in the wrong place, separated from mother, they have defensive behaviors which may cause changes to brain wiring that are harmful in the future. Severe stress without a parent to support her can be toxic to the newborn's brain.

The premature baby is not in an incubator because she is unstable, she is unstable because she is in an incubator! *N. Bergman 2004*

Babies should not need to cry.

Premies should never cry.

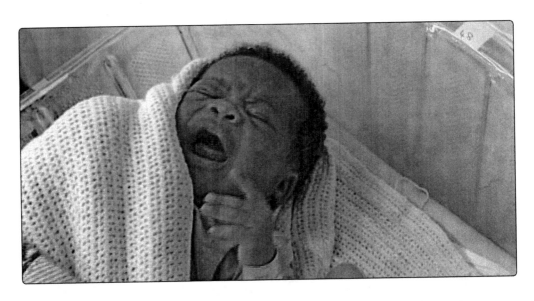

Protest:

When a baby is separated from her mother, her safe place, her response is often to cry. Crying is the baby's way of communicating with her mom to pick her up (1), feed her, soothe her or change her nappy. Crying is also her protest that she is alone and frightened. Her arms and legs move to get mom's attention (2).

Hard crying also forces open a valve between the two parts of the heart, so that blood without oxygen is sent to the brain instead of the lungs (3). It is dangerous for the brain to be without oxygen.

The premie's brain feels unsafe and releases stress hormones like cortisol which increase her heart rate, blood pressure and speeds up her breathing. If you imagine the blood vessels carrying blood from the heart to the brain, they are like a tree trunk. These vessels make thinner branches and eventually tiny "twigs" called capillaries. When the baby cries a lot, the blood pressure and volume increases too much in these tiny vessels. They may burst causing a bleed in the "ventricles", which are spaces in the middle of the brain where spinal fluid is made (4).

Stress will be seen in the baby's body as it makes her back arch and her legs and arms move a lot. This uses up a lot of energy which the baby should be using to grow.

Stress will release the hormone somatostatin which inhibits growth hormone and prevents the stomach from absorbing food effectively (5). Somatostatin and cortisol can stay in the body for up to an hour after crying.

> **Stress will affect the emotions and mind of the baby; as she will think that "nobody hears me crying or cares that I am alone and frightened".**
> **In the brain, there is "hyper-arousal" or vigilance (6).**

Despair:

If the baby cries for a long time she becomes exhausted, and runs out of calories; because of that she stops crying. At this stage, despair sets in. It is a more dangerous stage of the defense program. In this time, the stress hormones are still circulating, trying to speed up the body (for a "fight or flight" reaction to danger). But at the same time her brain sends nerve signals to slow down the body to save energy. The baby's brain does not know how to cope with these opposite messages (7)!

Her heart rate slows by ten beats per minute and her temperature goes down by more than 1°F to conserve energy for as long as possible in the hope that her mother will come back. Her breathing may become irregular, she moves less and her body is still. This state does look like sleep and rest, but it may in fact be "defensive freeze", which can be followed by "dissociation' (this is a typical reptile defense).

The baby feels abandoned and withdraws into herself.

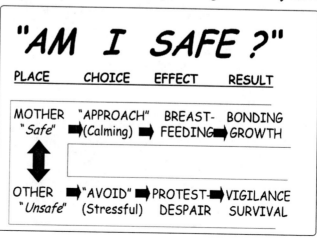

"AM I SAFE?"

PLACE	CHOICE	EFFECT	RESULT
MOTHER "Safe" ⟶	"APPROACH" (Calming) ⟶	BREAST-FEEDING ⟶	BONDING GROWTH
⇕			
OTHER "Unsafe" ⟶	"AVOID" (Stressful) ⟶	PROTEST- DESPAIR ⟶	VIGILANCE SURVIVAL

Research has shown that these babies have increased activity in the avoidance center of the brain. When this happens a lot, her brain-wiring will make her distrust people and be emotionally distant; she may have trouble bonding later (8).

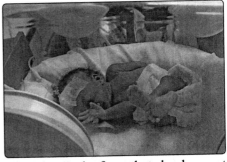

A tiny baby has not yet developed a separate sense of self. Her very being is connected to her mother for the first months of life. When a tiny baby is separated from her mother she goes through what psychologists call "annihilation anxiety", she fears that she does not exist, or that she will die (9).

This is why a baby reacts so strongly to being separated from her mother.

> **A baby needs to be held by her mother for physical and emotional well-being.**

For a preterm baby this separation is even more frightening. The premie should be developing and maturing in the womb, "a designer milieu". Instead, she may suddenly find herself in a noisy NICU with bright lights and the sharp noises of beeping machines. Worst of all, she is separated from her mother! Imagine what this does to her developing brain! This may in fact be the direct cause of the long term physical and emotional problems that premies are at higher risk of acquiring. This tiny brain is now brain-wiring for a life that it expects to be stressful (10). The defense pathways become this baby's way of coping with stress instead of calmer thinking and trusting. In this situation, the baby is wary and alert, and at risk for developing high blood pressure later in life (11). Not having food when she is hungry makes her body store food more, and she may tend to obesity and diabetes when she is grown up. (8;12)

How can you tell if your baby is in protest or despair? She will show small signs that say "stop" or "give me a break" or "help me to calm down". Learn to recognize the specific signs of your own baby being "disorganized".

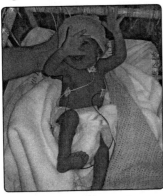

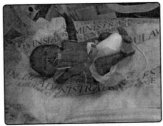

Sitting on air (protest)
Arms extended

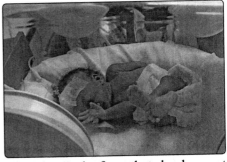

Looking away
(gaze aversion)

Stop sign (protest)

> **Watch your own baby carefully and respond to her messages.**

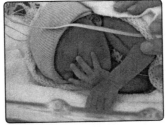

Hiding face (despair)

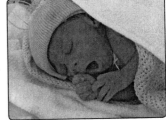

Yawning (despair)

These are some of the signs of a baby who is stressed and disorganized:

This list may be oversimplified, but may help you to recognize some of the signs. Place a check next to which signs you have seen when your own baby is upset.

Protest

- ☐ She cries.
- ☐ She holds her breath – apnea.
- ☐ Her heart rate increases.
- ☐ Her blood pressure increases.
- ☐ Her skin color becomes red, darkens or becomes blotchy.
- ☐ She extends or stretches her arms and legs out sideways.
- ☐ She arches her back stiffly.
- ☐ She spreads her arms out wide and holds them stiffly.
- ☐ She splays her fingers and toes.
- ☐ She puts her hands in front of her face with a 'stop sign'.
- ☐ Her movements are jerky and there are twitches or tremors.
- ☐ She "sits on air" with her legs up in the air at right angles to her body.
- ☐ She fusses and squirms.
- ☐ She sneezes, hiccups and spits up.

Despair

- ☐ Her breathing is irregular.
- ☐ Her heart rate decreases.
- ☐ Her oxygen saturation decreases.
- ☐ She looks away from you.
- ☐ She becomes limp.
- ☐ She yawns.
- ☐ She frowns.
- ☐ Small twitches of face muscles and fingers.

How to calm a distressed baby

If your premie is showing signs of protest or despair, she is in distress and needs you! Ideally, she wants to be picked up and held in skin-to-skin contact. For ANY baby you can gently place your hand over her body and hold your hand still. You can also cup one hand around her head and one around her feet to contain her. Flex her legs and bring her hand or fist next to her mouth. This will give her security. Help your baby to find ways to keep herself calm. This is called "self-soothing" or "self-regulating".

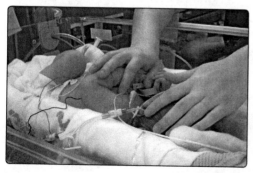 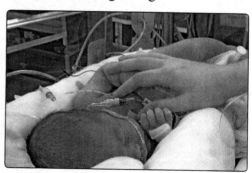

Do ***not*** rock her or shake or jig her up and down or pat her back.

The next chapter on developmental care will give you more help on how to avoid stress for your baby.

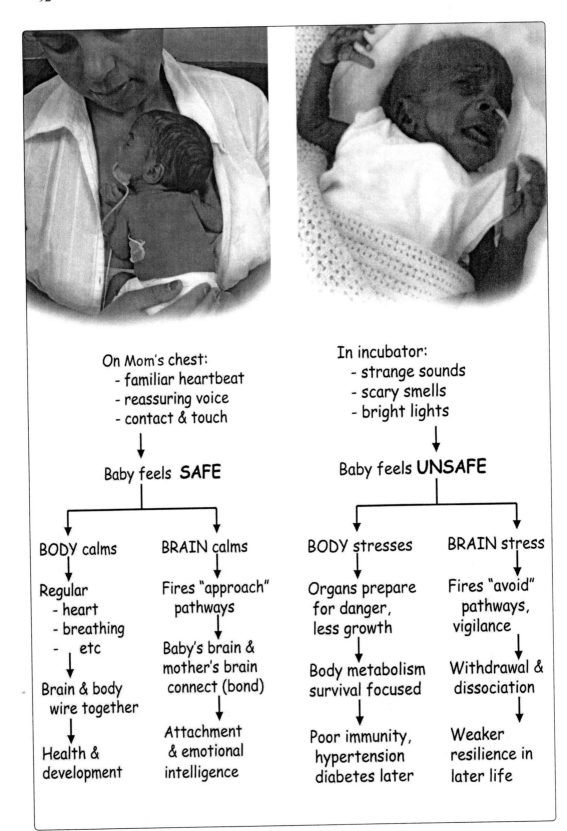

On Mom's chest:
- familiar heartbeat
- reassuring voice
- contact & touch

↓

Baby feels **SAFE**

BODY calms

Regular
- heart
- breathing
- etc

↓

Brain & body wire together

↓

Health & development

BRAIN calms

Fires "approach" pathways

↓

Baby's brain & mother's brain connect (bond)

↓

Attachment & emotional intelligence

In incubator:
- strange sounds
- scary smells
- bright lights

↓

Baby feels **UNSAFE**

BODY stresses

Organs prepare for danger, less growth

↓

Body metabolism survival focused

↓

Poor immunity, hypertension diabetes later

BRAIN stress

Fires "avoid" pathways, vigilance

↓

Withdrawal & dissociation

↓

Weaker resilience in later life

Fine Print Page – Separation and Stress

1. Separation distress calls are universal among mammals, including humans! Quote: "this cry is not dependent on earlier social experience and may be a genetically encoded reaction to separation".

2. This article describes the actual brain circuits in the parents that are activated by the above distress call, quote: "networks of highly conserved hypothalamic-midbrain-limbic-paralimbic-cortical circuits act in concert to support aspects of parent response to infants". These make parents "generally compelled to approach a crying infant … Infant cry–care loops may thus be thought of as part of an elaborate, dynamic and interactive com-munication system that maintains proximity to and elicits care from caregivers".

3. Summarizes many adverse effects, and identifies skin-to-skin contact as effective care!

4. This is an old, but original study that showed effect of crying, opening the foramen ovale, with right to left shunting, as seen in the fetus.

5. Somatostatin "lowers the rate of gastric emptying, reduces smooth muscle contractions and blood flow within the intestine. Collectively, has the overall effect of decreasing the rate of nutrient absorption." http://www.vivo.colostate.edu/hbooks/pathphys/endocrine/otherendo/somatostatin.html

6. Perry describes responses to threat, the first of which is vigilance, then freeze, finally dissociation.

7. Schore describes these in slightly different terms, (hyperarousal), with detail on the neuroanatomy. Quote: "... rapid alterations of ANS sympathetic ergotropic hyperarousal and parasympathetic trophotropic hy-poarousal create chaotic biochemical alterations, a toxic neurochemistry in the developing brain."

8. Teicher describes the neuronal and anatomical changes that abuse and neglect makes in the brain, but importantly suggests that these are adaptations to make the brain cope better in harsh world. But this adaptation is actually "maladaptive" in the social arena.

9. Hofer shows that early experiences do in fact impact on the quality of attachment. Quote: "behavioral, physiological and neural processes underlie the psychological constructs of attachment theory. It has become appar-ent that the unique features of early infant attachment reflect certain unique features of early infant sensory and mo-tor integration, early learning, communication, motivation and the regulation of biobehavioral sys-tems by the mother–infant interaction."

10. Pain is one of the main experiences of premies, and Anand describes some known consequences. Quote: "Perina-tal brain plasticity increases the vulnerability to early adverse experiences, thus leading to abnormal development and behavior."

11. This book describes the latest research field: epigenetics, whereby we now have clearer understanding of the mechanisms of how environment and experience change the brain and the body.

12. Barker was the first to identify such effects, looking at babies born with low-birth weight. He described a "thrifty phenotype" with altered metabolism leading to obesity and hypertension, and later diabetes.

Reference List

(1) Christensson K, Cabrera T, Christensson E, Uvnas-Moberg K, Winberg J. Separation distress call in the hu-man neonate in the absence of maternal body contact. Acta Paediatr 1995 May;84(5):468-73.

(2) Swain JE, Lorberbaum JP, Kose S, Strathearn L. Brain basis of early parent-infant interactions: psychology, physiology, and in vivo functional neuroimaging studies. Journal of Child Psychology & Psychiatry 2007 March;48(3/4):262-87.

(3) Ludington-Hoe SM, Cong X, Hashemi F. Infant crying: nature, physiologic consequences, and select inter-ven-tions. Neonatal Network: NN 2002 March;21(2):29-36.

(4) Lind J. Changes in the circulation and lungs at birth. Acta Paediatrica Supplementum 1960 March;49 (Suppl 122):39-52.

(5) Widstrom AM, Marchini G, Matthiesen AS, Werner S, Winberg J, Uvnas-Moberg K. Nonnutritive sucking in tube-fed preterm infants: effects on gastric motility and gastric contents of somatostatin. J Pediatr Gastroen-terol Nutr 1988 July;7(4):517-23.

(6) Perry BD, Pollard RA, Blakely TL, Baker WL, Vigilante D. Childhood trauma, the neurobiology of adaptation and "use-dependent" development of the brain. How"states" become "traits". Infant Mental health 1995;16(4):271-91.

(7) Schore AN. The effects of early relational trauma on right brain development, affect regulation, and infant mental health. Infant Mental Health Journal 2001;22(1-2):201-69.

(8) Teicher MH, Andersen SL, Polcari A, Anderson CM, Navalta CP. Developmental neurobiology of childhood stress and trauma. Psychiatr Clin North Am 2002 June;25(2):397-426.

(9) Hofer MA. The psychobiology of early attachment. Clinical Neuroscience Research 2005;XX:1-10.

(10) Anand KJ, Scalzo FM. Can adverse neonatal experiences alter brain development and subsequent behavior? Biology Of The Neonate 2000 February;77(2):69-82.

(11) Gluckman P, Hanson M. The Fetal Matrix Evolution, Development and Disease. The Press Syndicate of the University of Cambridge; 2005.

(12) Barker DJ. In utero programming of chronic disease. Clinical Science (London, England: 1979) 1998 Au-gust;95(2):115-28.

DEVELOPMENTAL CARE

> **Things you do now for your premie can make a huge difference later.**

You, her parents, are her SAFE place! BE THERE! GET INVOLVED!

> **Premies are very small and very sensitive; they sense everything!**

Protect your baby's senses.

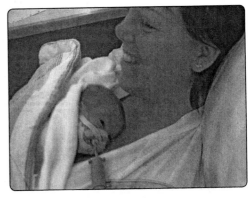

- ☐ Touch: Skin-to-Skin Contact should start from birth, or as soon as possible. Hold your baby firmly, close, still and contained and she will be calmer to grow faster. Handle her gently; flex her legs and arms with her hands near her mouth.

- ☐ Smell: your baby longs for the smell of your breast and your breastmilk; avoid strongly perfumed soap.

- ☐ Taste: your baby should taste your breastmilk.

The best developmental care – on mom.

- ☐ Sound: your premie knows your voice, speak to her!

- ☐ Sight: your baby can recognize your face.

Respond as soon as she shows signs of discomfort and before her body has becomes severely stressed or sick.

Nest and position her in the incubator to support her developing muscles.

> **WATCH YOUR INDIVIDUAL BABY AND LEARN WHAT UPSETS HER.**
> **Fix or change what you can.**

Your premie is aware and has feelings. Talk to her as a person and tell her what you are going to do. She must never be treated like an object.

Modern technology can keep smaller and younger babies alive, but we want these babies to have the best <u>quality</u> of life as well, so we have to treat them extra gently. Her brain needs to be protected from stress as it is very fragile.

"Developmental Care" is a term used by many people and can mean many different things. Here I am using the term Developmental Care to mean a gentle method of caring for all babies, especially for the premature baby, which will support the healthy development of body, brain and emotions by minimizing stress, and so reducing problems for the baby in the future.

Mom and Dad, your premie baby was expecting another few weeks of being held curled up, warm, quiet, safe and protected, and being fed continuously in the womb. Now she has been born early, and lies in a noisy, busy, bright NICU. What a shock these changes must be for her!! No wonder she is frightened, cries and is unstable!

As you can see from the table below, holding your baby in Skin-to-Skin Contact makes her feel as if she is back in the womb and restores her to her safe place!

In Mom's womb baby expects	In incubator, baby experiences	On Mom's chest in skin-to-skin
Arms bent	Arms stick out sideways	Arms bent
Legs bent or flexed	Legs often extended	Legs bent or flexed
Quiet and peaceful sounds	Noisy, busy NICU, alarms	Quiet and peaceful sounds
Feels contained in mom	No containment, no boundaries	Mom's arms contain her
Back curled	Lies flat on back	Back curled
Fed continuously	Fed 2-4 hourly	Fed frequently
Nearly dark in womb	Bright lights	Gentle light inside shirt
Feels SAFE	Feels unsafe/frightened and alone	Feels SAFE
Mom's womb holds her	Handled by many nurses & doctors	Mom's arms hold her

Up to now, developmental care has been something that nurses in a NICU do to help a baby in an incubator. But as the major stress for tiny babies is to be separated from mother, a premie separated from her mother often struggles to stabilize herself or "self-regulate". **Without YOU, your baby cannot keep her stress levels down.**

I want to encourage you <u>both</u> to be with your baby, and to be aware of things that you can do to help your baby to regulate and be stable. You can support her so that she does not feel overwhelmed. She needs Skin-to-Skin Contact to help her physically; to keep her heart rate, breathing, blood pressure and temperature stable. She also needs Skin-to-Skin Contact to calm her down emotionally (1). Developmental care does not need to cost a lot of money.

Placing the premie in Skin-to-Skin Contact on mother's chest is the single most cost-effective "developmental care" change that we need to make in modern NICU's.

> **Our challenge will be to take the best of modern technology available to a premie and add it in the right place, on mother's chest.**

Ten years ago, incubator care was standard care for preterm babies. This is changing! There is no science proving the safety of incubators, but there is science showing the benefits of baby being on her mom's chest. Every hospital strives to provide ideal care for their patients within their understanding, but they need a specific focus of best care for brain growth, not just for physical survival. The key is Skin-to-Skin Contact. Here, all the developmental care essentials come together, as the baby feels safe. There are no stress hormones; she does not waste energy and can grow faster. She is held securely, and contained; she moves with mom, as she has done in the womb. Her physical development can be good and now you can add mental, emotional and social development!

All this works together to encourage secure attachment (1).

As we discussed in the neuroscience chapter, it is sensations which fire and wire the brain (see page 77). You want to give your baby the expected and familiar sensations that are going to make her feel safe. This feeling of being safe determines how your baby behaves. If she feels safe she will grow well.

Separation from you makes her stressed and you want to avoid stress.

> **Being on your chest in Skin-to-Skin Contact will make your baby feel safe.**

A picture of Developmental Care could be like looking at ripples in a pond. The very inside circle means giving the best care by handling each individual baby gently to support her own body systems to self-regulate. Physically this means stabilizing her heart rate, breathing, blood pressure and temperature. Emotionally this is seen as keeping her calmer and unstressed. The next ripple would be looking how we can make her most comfortable, on mother or in an incubator, so we look at her bed or nest. Then we look at her incubator, then into the larger external NICU ward environment by reducing noise and light to reduce stress, save her energy and help her grow. As she leaves the NICU she will still be small and sensitive and need "Developmental Care" awareness relating to her room and your home. As she grows stronger she will move out into wider society.

Some hospitals work with NIDCAP (Neonatal Individualized Developmental Care and Assessment Program). This is an advanced, structured developmental care program. NIDCAP carefully watches how each individual baby copes, and recommends detailed improvements in care (2;3).

A recent article shows that babies cared for in this way (NIDCAP) stabilize quicker. They have less chronic lung disease; they need less ventilation, less CPAP and less extra oxygen. They also go home sooner. It is also cost-effective as hospital stays are shorter. The babies have higher brain development scores at 9 and 12 months. At 18 months' adjusted age, they have less disability, especially less mental delay (10% compared to 30% on standard care) (4).

What can you do to help your preterm baby in the incubator?

There are times and stages when your baby needs to be in the incubator. I will suggest here some different ways which together will calm her. Restore the womb environment as much as possible.

You, Mom and Dad, will want to work to achieve best possible development for your baby. We may never know fully how the brain works and heals, but at least we can say that we did the best possible at the time.

What you can do to help your premie will depend on where she is.

Is she in labor ward?

Is she in the NICU?

How long has she been in NICU?

Does the NICU insist on using incubators?

Is she in a high tech, well-resourced hospital?

Is she in a low tech clinic?

Is a nurse or midwife with her, or is a doctor deciding on care?

What are the hospital policies on breastfeeding, Skin-to-Skin Contact, etc?

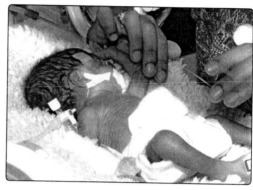

Now, parents and medical personnel can work together to help premies to survive with a better <u>quality</u> of life, physically and emotionally. For the doctor or nurse working in a NICU this will be their full time job, but they change duties every 8 or 12 hours. You are your premie's Mom and Dad, and you are the only possible constant support she has. Your touch, your smell, your voices and faces are most important for your baby. The small things that you do now can have a hugely positive impact on your baby's long term development. Understanding the biology behind the development is important.

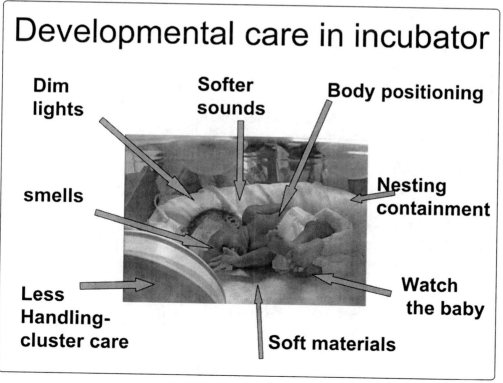

Developmental care in incubator

Dim lights

Softer sounds

Body positioning

smells

Nesting containment

Less Handling-cluster care

Soft materials

Watch the baby

Every NICU is different; there will be parts of the NICU that are wonderful. Appreciate those and encourage the staff members. There will also be some things which you will want to improve on now that you know the neuroscience.

We will look at each sensation in detail:

Touch (this includes, touching, holding, contact, carrying and moving your baby).

The sense of touch develops early inside the mother. The baby inside you has constant pressure from the amniotic fluid.

There are two pathways for touch –

- **deep physical contact or "containment" is calming**
- **and light (feather) touch stimulates or irritates.**

Deep physical contact or "containment" is continued contact and pressure on the body. When you hold your baby in Skin-to-Skin Contact firmly, close and still, you calm your baby and reassure her that she is safe. This is essential for your tiny premie. Her brain development can continue closer to normal and Skin-to-Skin Contact helps her to develop good muscle tone. Carrying your premie tied on your chest in Skin-to-Skin Contact with her airway stabilized is the best for your premie. Her legs should be flexed and her hands should be near her mouth so that she can comfort herself.

When you need to move her, do so slowly, and turn her over so her back is up, pausing if she gets stressed. Keep her arms and legs contained as you move her.

Light touch or stroking the skin with feather touch is arousing, and irritates your premie as she is unable to screen out all the messages that she receives. Premies are fragile and do not like to be stroked lightly. (Few adults like to have a spider crawling on them, but everyone needs a firm hug!) If your baby has an apnea attack or stops breathing, then the arousing is good as light stroking may stimulate her to breathe.

Your baby's skin is very thin and sensitive; remember to use soft natural fibers with a close weave and avoid rough towels.

Contain her arms and legs and hold her still.

Touching your baby if she is in the incubator

In the past, parents were not allowed to touch their premies in the incubator. Understanding the two different touch sensations is the key. Premies benefit from pressure touch, they do not like light feather touch. Keep an eye on the monitors, and watch her stabilize as you place your hands over her. Human touch is essential for your baby.

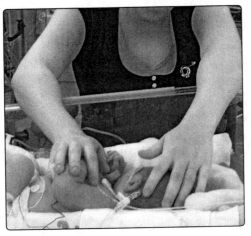

Your premie in the NICU will be handled by very many nurses and doctors, often with painful injections or putting tubes down her throat, etc. Mom and Dad, do try to be there to calm your baby when she is becoming stressed .You can buffer the pain by your holding her during these painful procedures. You as parents are the primary care-givers, and nurses are there to teach and support you.

Wash your hands for 2 minutes with unperfumed soap before every contact with your infant. Start by placing your hands firmly and gently over her body. This will help her feel contained and safe. Hold your hands still. It can also be helpful to cup one hand around the top of her head and one hand around her feet or bottom.

Ask the nurses to teach you how to move your baby. Place your hands over her body and hold her legs and arms close to her body so that her body is moved as a whole without her arms flopping out sideways. This will help her vestibular system, which is important for balance.

You can also try putting your little finger in her palm. She may well grasp it. This is her lifeline to help pull her through these long weeks. From 35 weeks onwards, infant massage can help, but be sensitive to her reactions.

Nesting and positioning

In your womb, your baby had firm, soft and flexible boundaries. She was curled up in the "fetal position" with her legs together and flexed, and with her arms bent and her hands near her mouth. She has probably been sucking her thumb for a long time as this is self-soothing.

When your baby is born prematurely, the ideal is to restore her to the same fetal position.

> **Hold her in a fetal position with her legs and arms curled up.**

If your baby has to stay in the incubator she is often not strong enough to make herself comfortable and she lies with her legs and arms "extended" or stretched out and often "floppy". It is important to position and flex her by making a tight nest with firm, soft, flexible boundaries with rolls of cloth so that she can lie curled up in the fetal position in the incubator. This flexed position helps her to feel secure and contained. The nest

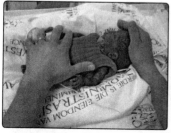
Place your hands over her, hold still. Contain her arms & legs.

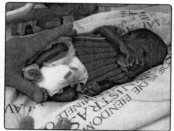
Bend legs & give feet a boundary to press against.

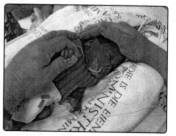
Cup hands around her head, contain arm, let her hold your finger.

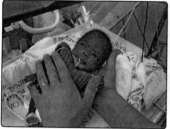
Moving of premie: hand over body to contain her. Pause if she shows signs of stress.

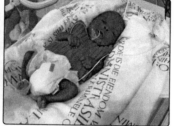
Make a tight nest to contain her.

> **Nesting**
> **and**
> **Positioning**

should curl her shoulders forward; keep her arms near the midline and her hips to the centre. Help her lie on her side, and sometimes on her tummy. Your baby will need a close boundary to push her feet against.

Over time, positioning affects your baby's development. A premie often lies in an incubator for 6–10 weeks and long-term damage can be done which will cause her problems later on. This can be avoided by correct positioning in the NICU. (See page 124, the long-term problems chapter.)

Your premie has very soft bones and should have been developing in the amniotic fluid inside the womb where she would be less affected by gravity. As she has not finished developing, her head can easily become flattened if she lies on her back all the time. By moving your baby's head position even a little bit so that she lies on all sides of the head, her head will stay more rounded. If she stays in the same position for long periods, flat on her back in NICU, she becomes stiff in the shoulders and hips which may cause problems later.

Warmth

> **When your baby is held in Skin-to-Skin Contact, she will have a much more even temperature than if she were in an incubator.**

Mother's skin has a comforting constant temperature. An incubator heats at one time and cools at another so the temperature is always changing.

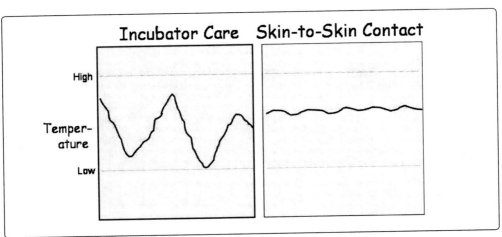

Smell

> **Smell is one of the strongest senses at birth so she can find the breast and feed to survive.**

Your smell will be familiar to her from the amniotic fluid, so she will be reassured and calm. Smelling your breast will encourage early breastfeeding. One of the many benefits of Skin-to-Skin Contact is that normal stomach hormones are released. Her stomach works better, absorbing all the food and this helps her to grow faster. Avoid wearing strong deodorants or perfume. Shower daily and wash your hands regularly (5).

If she is in the incubator some hospitals will insist on alcohol gel, or other antiseptics for your hands. These smell unpleasant to a premie. Wait until they evaporate before touching your baby.

If you are not able to hold her, ask if you can take a small soft facecloth or a piece of soft cotton and sleep with it, and then bring it into her incubator. That way she can smell you even when you are not there and this might soothe her (5;6).

Taste

> **Your baby is expecting to taste your breastmilk.**

We have looked at how breastmilk has the RIGHT and essential nutrients for growth, and how it varies in a wonderful way to give the premie exactly what she needs for completing her development (see page 58). But taste as a sensation is important for its brain wiring effects, not just for body growth.

Suckling gives your baby a sensation of the nipple and the breast itself. This sensation relaxes your baby; it pulls the nipple onto the top of the mouth (upper palate). This is a soothing centre, and releases hormones for digestion. Sucking on a pacifier can cause many problems with teeth growth and speech later. Even so, a pacifier might be better than leaving a baby to cry!

If your premie is in an incubator, she should still be given your breastmilk.

Sound

Inside you, your baby was already hearing by 23 weeks gestational age. The ear sends messages to the brain. Sounds can all be heard, but they are all muffled by mom's body. She can already recognize your voices. Sound is tied to day/night rhythms and movement. From 30 weeks onwards, babies like quiet voices with changing rhythms (7).

> **Your baby cannot shut her ears to loud sounds and feels them as pain.**

When she is born, keep noise levels low. Newborns listen simultaneously to everything and cannot screen out sounds. You will learn to pick up your child's individual sensitivity. She will react to some sounds badly and not to others.

Some mothers have found that their child settles when hearing a tape recording of her voice talking or singing. This does not work for all babies, but may be worth a try.

If your baby is in an incubator and you are feeling helpless sitting next to her, talk, read and sing to her. Your voice will calm her (8).

> **Do not drop things or tap on top of the incubator!**
> **Close incubator doors slowly and quietly.**

The entire incubator box can become a resonance chamber which magnifies sound.

The NICU should be kept as quiet as possible. Some NICUs have a sound meter to remind people to keep the noise levels low. Mobile phones should preferably be switched off (or on silent) and voices kept quiet.

Simply dimming the lights encourages people to speak more quietly.

Sight

Before 30 weeks gestational age, a premie is not able to constrict her pupils to limit the amount of light coming into her eyes. This only works properly after about 34 weeks. Before 32 weeks, the eyelids also do not limit the entry of light. We therefore need to protect the premie's developing eyes from direct light exposure (9).

Your premature baby's eyes are very sensitive to light. Keep lights dim.

When she is on your chest with "tummy to mommy" with your shirt and blankets over you both, her eyes will be protected.

We also need to protect your premie's REM sleep (see page 83, the sleep cycling section). Your baby needs periods of darkness or low light in the NICU to help her regulate her own biological clock and get her day/night rhythm in place. Natural light is far better than artificial light, and fluorescent lights are worse for her, they are too bright and they flicker. Switch off lights not in use.

If she is in the incubator put dark covers on her eyes or place a dark cloth over the incubator. You may find she sleeps better simply by laying her down facing away from bright windows.

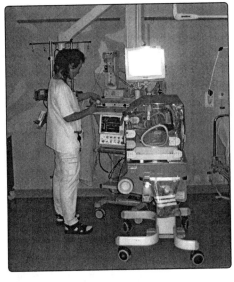

If your baby needs phototherapy, check that she has very dark, soft eye covers to protect her eyes, covering around the edges as well.

Individual personality or sensitivity

It is very important to remember that each baby is a wonderful individual with her own personality. Your own baby is unique, with her own likes and dislikes! She will react to things differently from another baby (2,3).

Watch your baby to see what she can do and support that; see what she cannot do, and help her. Look for her competence. Some babies can breathe on their own at 28 weeks gestational age, others can't. Some can co-ordinate sucking, swallowing and breastfeeding, while others at the same age need help.

"Behavior of the infant is its primary way to communicate."
– Dr Heidelise Als

Watch your baby, especially her face, to pick up her own unique messages to you, which tell you how she is feeling. Read the small signs of your own baby being "disorganized"; signs that say "stop" or "give me a break" or "help me to calm down". If you are watching your baby in the incubator and can pick up the little signals of stress and respond to her quickly, you will help her to avoid becoming unstable or sick. Help her to self-regulate or find her balance by placing your hands on her and holding her still. You will know her better than anybody as you will spend hours watching her (10).

Premature babies are fragile and sensitive, and will show their stress in different ways. Different babies react differently to stimulation. Some are more sensitive and will quickly be overwhelmed. Mom, you will need to be sensitive to your baby's responses to you; be respectful and stop doing anything if she is becoming stressed (11).

> **If your premie is showing stress signals: stop and hold her still until her body calms down and she settles, her heart rate is normal and her body is still.**

"Clustering care", which means doing all procedures together with minimal handling, means that your baby can get longer rest times, and good sleep cycling. You can help her keep balanced by lovingly watching her carefully to see what she can cope with.

A good general idea for premies is to do only ONE thing at a time at first. For example, if your baby was born at 32 weeks gestation, let her look at you, but don't talk at the same time. This may over-stimulate her. Give her small doses of stimulation and stop if she looks away or shows any of the stress signals. In time, she will cope with lots of messages at once. "Stop" – doing whatever has upset her – even talking to her or making eye contact can be too much for her. "Look" around – are there bright lights that may be hurting her eyes? "Listen" for loud noises that may have disturbed her.

> **Watch your baby!**

See the signs of a baby who is stressed and disorganized in the Separation & Stress chapter (see page 91).

If your baby's oxygen level drops ("desaturation"), it can be bad for her brain. This happens with apnea (baby stops breathing) and with bradycardia (heart slows down). These usually come together. If this happens, tickling her and doing the feather touching may arouse her, but the same touching may have caused it! Often more vigorous stimulation is required to start the breathing and get the heart rate up. To prevent this, do not handle her a lot. Calm containing and holding will help, however. Don't change nappies if she is upset and restless.

Don't watch the monitors – watch your little person. She needs you to learn to read her signals and to change what you do to make her feel better.

For example, if she gets unsettled or unstable when you are tube-feeding her, slow down the speed of flow of the milk.

If she is uncomfortable after a feed, maybe her tummy is too full (like you after a big dinner). Give her less milk at a time – remember her tiny stomach is only the size of a marble – and feed her more often.

Questions about your NICU

Light

Does your NICU have bright lights or dim? ....

Are the lights dimmed at night to help your baby get a day/night rhythm? ....

Can you place a dark cloth over the incubator? ....

Noise

Is the NICU full of loud noises? ....

Are loud noises or mobile phones allowed? ....

Is there a noise monitor? ....

Is there an awareness of speaking softly and are there reminder charts? ....

Here are some things to look for in your baby – find your own too.

What makes her cry?	
Does her body jerk when there is a loud sound?	
Does she react to bright light?	
Is she unsettled after she has eaten?	
What makes your baby's oxygen level drop? (desaturation)	
What makes her scrunch up her face unhappily?	
What things that happen in the NICU does she react badly to?	
Does she react to strong smells?	
Does she turn towards your voice?	
Does she relax when you hold her close to you?	
When do her eyes open most?	
How does she react if you sing to her?	
What are her most calm and awake times during the day?	
How long can she interact with you before getting too tired?	
Does she like to lie on her side?	
Is she calmer if she is contained in a nest in the incubator?	
Does she sleep better on your chest or in the incubator?	
Is her breathing more regular when she is lying flat or up at an angle?	

Look for these signs showing that your baby is peaceful.

Her arms and legs are curled up in the flexed, fetal position.

Her heart rate, breathing and oxygen saturation are even.

Her skin color is even.

Her face looks relaxed.

Her eyes open.

Her hands are near her face.

She may suck on her fist.

Her hands are gently curled up and may be clasped together.

She may hold on to your finger.

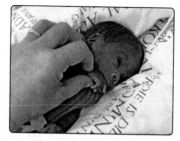

Contain arm + finger hold.

Maybe you could work with the nurses to put up a list of things on her incubator that your baby is sensitive to.

There are differences between premies born at different stages. These differences depend on how prematurely your baby was born (the gestational age). Remember that each baby is an individual, so she may be 32 weeks, but can be small for her age, or weaker. Here are three broad groups with some ideas for care.

Read whichever applies to your baby!

Near term (more than 36 weeks)

At nearly fullterm, babies are usually reasonably strong and able to cope without extra technology. The best care for them would be Skin-to-Skin Contact. This Skin-to-Skin Contact will help breastfeeding to start immediately after birth, and the baby will be warm with a stable heart rate when she is on her mother. Avoiding separation is the best care.

Premature (32 – 36 weeks)

These babies are usually reasonably stable, and usually do well without lots of machinery. The premie is usually strong enough and developed enough to start breastfeeding straight after delivery. She can suck and swallow safely. Your premie will need your Skin-to-Skin Contact to keep her temperature, heart rate and oxygen saturation stable. She will grow twice as fast in Skin-to-Skin Contact compared to incubator care. Avoid separation by doing as much Skin-to-Skin Contact as you can. This provides the best stability for her development and brain wiring.

Skin-to-Skin Contact can still be done with all the monitors attached. The NICU nurses can help you to transfer the baby safely.

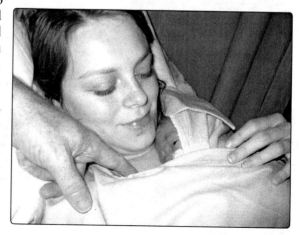

Very premature (<32w)

In Skin-to-Skin Contact

If your baby is less than 32 weeks, her lungs are maybe not developed enough to breathe yet and she may need technical support. You can still do Skin-to-Skin Contact with all the machinery, but the staff of your NICU will need to be experienced to do this. By keeping all the monitors attached during Skin-to-Skin Contact, you and the staff will see how stable baby is. This will give an objective measure of how well she is coping.

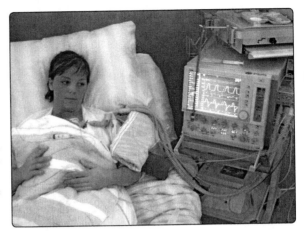

In the incubator

Her brain still has a lot of developing to do, and you want to help your fragile tiny baby. Under 28 weeks of gestation the number of problems premies face is very much greater. Importantly, here you need to avoid her crying which increases blood pressure and places her at increased risk of a brain bleed. Also, do not lift her feet too high when you change her diaper.

Do all you can with "developmental care" to help avoid stress for your premie. Being next to her and putting your hand on her back in the incubator may be all you can do for her at this stage, but she really needs you to be there with her. Talk gently to her.

Importantly, the lights should be dimmed, as her pupils cannot constrict. Positioning and nesting are important (12).

Little things done early can make a huge difference later!

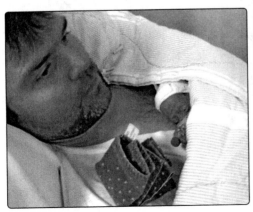

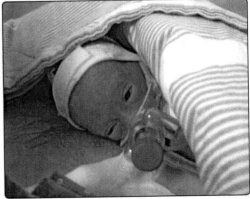

Fine Print Page – Developmental care

All of these references are recommended reading, and practical to apply in neonatal care.

1. This and some of the articles that follow on this page, come from a hard cover journal, all of which deals with sensory environment, which is core to development and subsequent attachment.
2. NIDCAP was developed by Heidelise Als. A key concept is involvement of the family.
3. Another key concept is that the framework (synactive model) is holistic. The positive outcome does not come from doing one or two things, like covering incubators or nesting, but from the "total care package".
4. This is the largest study on NIDCAP to date, and provides a clear review of previous studies, and a good explanation of the principles of NIDCAP. It shows the improvement in long-term developmental care out-comes for premies given NIDCAP care.
5. Smell is far more important to the newborn than we realize!
6. The cloth idea might seem simplistic …and some may object to it being "unsterile"! Babies that get mom's milk have good immunity, and are calmed by her smell.
7. This article explains both the positive and harmful effects of sound in general,
8. Mother's voice is regulating: quote "The newborn shows heart rate decelerations in response to speech sounds. Early experience with voice has acute and enduring effects on the developing brain … with effects (on) development of the auditory system, as well as for later social and emotional development.."
9. Visual development is very complex … but one of the key aspects for the premature is ensuring sleep and protection from bright light, "Spontaneous synchronous retinal waves occur in preterm infants in the neona-tal intensive care unit and must be protected, as they are critical for visual development."
10. This is a very hands-on and practical article by one of the very first NIDCAP pioneers.
11. This book describes the stress behaviors in detail.
12. Another practical paper, identifies 16 better care practices and discusses the practical implementation of each in detail, "containment and body flexion" is the first. http://www.nature.com/jp/journal/v27/n2s/pdf/7211843a.pdf

Reference List

(1) Browne JV. Early relationship environments: physiology of Skin-to-Skin Contact for parents and their pre-term infants. Clin Perinatol 2004 June;31(2):287-98, vii.

(2) Als H, Butler S. Newborn individualized developmental care and assessment program (NIDCAP) . Changing the future for infants and families in intensive care nurseries. Early Childhood Services 2008;2(1):1-20.

(3) Als H. A synactive model of neonatal behavioral organization: framework for the assessment of neurobehav-ioral development in the premature infant and for support of infants and parents in the neonatal intensive care environment. Physical & Occupational Therapy in Pediatrics 1986;6(3/4):3-53.

(4) Peters KL, Rosychuk RJ, Hendson L, Cote JJ, McPherson C, Tyebkhan JM. Improvement of short-and long-term outcomes for very low birth weight infants: Edmonton NIDCAP trial. Pediatrics 2009;124:1009-20.

(5) Schaal B, Hummel T, Soussignan R. Olfaction in the fetal and premature infant: functional status and clinical implications. Clin Perinatol 2004 June;31(2):261-vii.

(6) Cernoch JM, Porter RH. Recognition of maternal axillary odors by infants. Child Dev 1985 December;56(6):1593-8.

(7) Gray L, Philbin MK. Effects of the neonatal intensive care unit on auditory attention and distraction. Clin Perinatol 2004 June;31(2):243-60.

(8) Fifer. W.P, Moon CM. The role of mother's voice in the organization of brain function in the newborn. Acta Paediatr 1994;Suppl 397:86-93.

(9) Graven SN. Early neurosensory visual development of the fetus and newborn. Clin Perinatol 2004 June;31(2):199-216, v.

(10) Lawhon G. Management of stress in premature infants. In: Angelini DJ, Whelan Knapp CM, Gibes RM, editors. Perinatal/Neonatal Nursing. A Clinical handbook. Boston: Blackwell Scientific Publications; 1986. p. 319-27.

(11) Madden SL. The preemie parents companion. Massachusetts: Harvard Common Press; 2000.

(12) Laudert S, Liu WF, Blackington S, Perkins B, Martin S, Millan-York E et al. Implementing potentially better practices to support the neurodevelopment of infants in the NICU. Journal of Perinatology 2007 December 2;27:S75-S93.

TECHNOLOGY

Mom and Dad, it is normal to feel overwhelmed by all of the machinery and monitors in the NICU at first, and you may feel helpless. The technology described in these pages is needed for your baby's survival, but she still needs you. You have the right to be with her, to be as close to her as possible, and to touch her, and then to hold her on your naked chest as soon as possible.

DO NOT BE SCARED OF THE MACHINES.

All of the machines may seem complicated and sophisticated, but the machines really do rather simple things and the basic concepts are NOT complicated. For each section in this chapter, there are some simple explanations and "buzzwords" or technical jargon and abbreviations. There is also a table of basics and a space for your doctor to explain and fill in what your baby needed.

NOTE to health professionals: for this chapter parents need help to fill in terms and explanation in appropriate words, space is provided!

Every baby is different but understanding the medical jargon may help you. The nurses and doctors often use abbreviations. You are allowed this information. You are her parents, so find out as much about the technology as you can. Find out about her needs and set about providing them – this makes it easier to cope and begins to empower you to care for your baby.

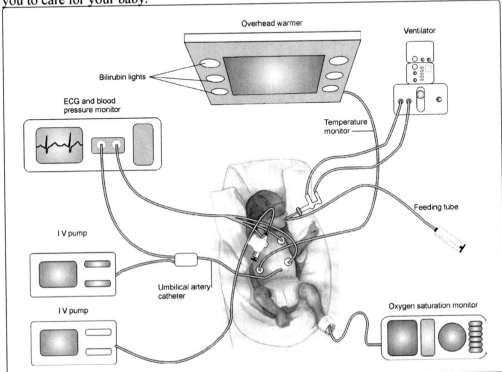

Your baby has been born early and now no longer gets food, blood circulation and oxygen via the umbilical cord, so she has to get her own systems going. Some of these may not yet be fully developed. The hospital staff will need to assess what she will need help with in terms of machinery or technology.

Resuscitation and birth period

At birth the staff will do an <u>APGAR score</u>, a 1–10 score of your baby's heart and lung condition. They will usually do this at 1, 5 and 10 minutes.

Your baby may need Cardio (heart) Pulmonary (lung) Resuscitation (CPR) to help to get the heart and lungs and breathing working. Sometimes they need to intubate (put a tube into your baby's lungs) to help her breathe. Sometimes babies are suctioned at birth. This is done less often these days, but it is done if there is fluid in the airways. The noise may sound worrying for parents.

<u>What resuscitation did your baby need?</u>

....

....

....

....

....

<u>Breathing and Oxygen</u>

Getting oxygen throughout the body needs three things:

> the heart to pump,
>
> the lungs to fill with air,
>
> and the hemoglobin in the blood to carry the oxygen to the body tissues.

Each of these can be supported.

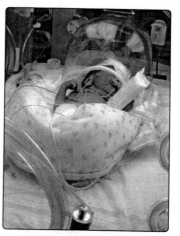

The fetus inside the mother gets her oxygen from the mother via the placenta from the mother's bloodstream. When the baby is born the baby's lungs have to fill with air. The very first breath she takes does this fully. She doesn't need to cry to do this.

The lungs may not be ready to inflate properly. Surfactant helps the lungs to inflate, but may not be enough in a premie. Steroids given to the mother two days before the birth will increase surfactant. The doctors may need to give artificial surfactant to the baby.

Baby under oxygen hood

Here is some of the technical help your preterm baby may need for breathing:

Abbreviations:	Translated	Meaning
CPR	Cardio Pulmonary Resuscitation	Heart-lung support, the baby may need emergency help to start her heart beating and lungs breathing.
IPPV	Intermittent Positive Pressure Ventilation	A ventilator helps the lungs, which are elastic, to inflate by blowing in air under pressure.
	Oscillator	A high frequency ventilator
O_2 sats SaO_2	Oxygen Saturation	Clip with a red light attached to her finger or toe for checking level of oxygen in the blood.
	Oxygen Hood	A hood to cover the baby's head and give higher oxygen concentration.
	Nasal cannula	Tiny pipe with holes going into the nostrils with extra oxygen.
CPAP	Continuous Positive Airways Pressure	Extra push of pressure to get oxygen to the blood.
	Surfactant	Acts like a type of soap to help the lungs to inflate properly. It keeps the lungs soft and elastic so they can easily open and close.
Your Baby?		

Heart and circulation

For a premie, the heart is usually competent.

The heart has already been pumping in the womb, but now some valves direct the blood in the big blood vessels of the heart to flow in a different direction. Inside you your baby would be getting oxygen dissolved in her blood through the placenta and the umbilical cord. Suddenly, her body has to try to get her own oxygen and her heart has to circulate it around her body.

Your baby may be linked to a heart monitor. Many parents of premies spend those first agonizingly long weeks in the NICU gazing at the monitors ready to react if the red light flashes.

Heart Rate (HR) – this is how fast the heart is beating to pump blood around the body. The heart rate needs to be fast enough to circulate oxygen and food. The heart rate of a tiny premie will be faster than an adult's and it may also be very irregular. Initially the range is 120–160. An irregular heart rate may be evidence of instability. Small changes in heart rate are normal. The heart rate is usually easy to measure.

Blood Pressure (BP) – this needs to be high enough to push the blood to the tissues, but not so high that it bursts the blood vessels. Blood pressure is more difficult to measure than the heart rate. Medicines can be used to increase or decrease the heart rate, and increase blood pressure, or to help the heart muscle itself.

HR	**Heart rate**	
	Bradycardia	Slow heart rate
	Tachycardia	Fast heart rate
BP	**Blood pressure**	
	hypotension	Low blood pressure
	hypertension	High blood pressure
Your Baby?		

Fluid management

To carry the oxygen we need blood which means fluids.

The fetus gets all her fluid from the placenta.

The newborn baby must drink.

The newborn premie cannot drink enough! (The premature baby CAN safely swallow as she has been swallowing amniotic fluids since 16 weeks gestation.)

When a full-term baby is born, she has 10% extra weight which is liquid. This liquid is to help the baby cope for the first two or three days until her mother's breastmilk has started flow properly. Newborns often lose weight during the first three days as they lose that extra fluid.

For the premature this early weight loss needs to be managed carefully as breastfeeding takes longer to get started.

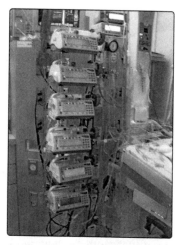
A baby may need all these drips

Premies are often unable to keep their fluid balance right. They lose a lot of fluid easily and dehydrate through the skin, so their body may need to be covered by a sheet of thin plastic to hold in the water. The air inside the incubator can be humidified to prevent evaporation loss. Skin-to-Skin Contact also prevents water loss through the skin.

The kidneys "clean" all the fluid in the body but they are only mature at 3 months after a full term birth.

Your baby may need a drip for fluids. This can be

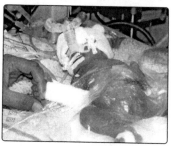
Baby's body covered in plastic.

placed in several ways (see "Lines" in the chart below). Various fluids can be given through these lines. You may be worried to find that your baby has a splint on the arm that has a drip. This is to stabilize the drip line, and does not mean that her arm is broken!

	Breastmilk	This is the best medicine any premature baby can be given!
	Neonatal maintenance solution	A carefully balanced liquid for premies.
TPN	**Total Parenteral Nutrition**	The tiny baby is fed into the veins, i.e. not through the stomach.
	a peripheral line	A drip directly into the veins of the hand, arm or foot or scalp.
	a central line	a tiny tube into a bigger vein, this lasts longer.
	an umbilical line	A drip put into the baby's umbilicus, this can be used for the first few days.
	arterial line	Sicker babies need to get fluid directly into the arteries
	enteral line	This tube goes straight into the stomach e.g. a naso-gastric tube – this is a good way to provide fluids.
Your Baby?		

Food management

In the womb, the baby would be getting exactly the right food from mom; it is dissolved in the blood in the placenta and carried to her in the umbilical cord. Inside mom, her stomach was working, but did not have much going through it. When your baby is born, she must eat and swallow for herself. Though her swallowing muscles are ready, the rest of her body may not be ready.

So she may need either a naso-gastric tube (NGT) into her nose or an oro-gastric tube (OGT) through her mouth straight into the stomach. The tube will be fixed to her face with tape and she will be given her food through it. Both NGT and OGT are sometimes called gavage feeding. Your expressed breastmilk is what she needs most to help her immunity to develop and to provide the food that her brain needs the most.

> **Your premie's gut is very immature. Actually, the gut is biologically immature until 6 months of age. Your baby's gut depends on human milk; mother's milk is protective. Any foreign substance can cause harm to the immature gut.**

Your baby needs a supply of brain fuel: this is critical. She also needs body fuel for her metabolism and she needs extra calories for growth. Your baby will have a growth chart in the NICU. In the first few days, her weight will probably go down a little. After this, you hope to see it going up. There may be dips now and then, but do not panic or be discouraged. Simple things may change: for example, was she weighed before or after a meal, before or after urinating, before a nappy change, or at a different time of day. There are many variables. Try to see the big trend.

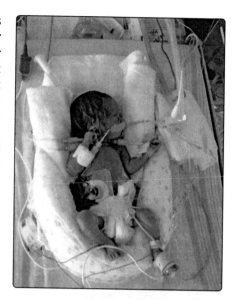

This baby has a 'stoma'

Abbreviations:	Translated	Meaning
EBM	Expressed Breastmilk:	the mother is encouraged to express or squeeze out or pump her breastmilk to be fed to her own baby.
MOM	Mothers own milk:	the best!
HMB	Human Milk Bank:	If a mother cannot supply milk, babies sometimes get pasteurized milk from other mothers.
AIF	Artificial Infant Formula:	dried cows' milk, with additives.
LC	Lactation Consultant:	someone specially trained to help with breastfeeding.
	Human Milk Fortifier:	Extra calories (sometimes with protein and minerals) to increase growth rate.
NGT	naso-gastric tube:	your baby will be given her liquid food or breastmilk through a tube going through her nose straight to her stomach.
OGT	oro-gastric tube:	your baby will be given her liquid food through a tube going through her mouth straight to her stomach.
	hypoglycemia:	low blood sugar level.

		hyperglycemia:	high blood sugar level.
Your Baby?			

Temperature management

In the mother's womb, the baby's body temperature is kept constant.

When the full term baby is born she needs to regulate her own temperature and can usually manage this. Above 5 lb, temperature control is usually good If the baby weighs less than 4 lb, the body mass is too small for the surface area and she cannot maintain her own temperature.

Even if the baby is bigger, a cold environment or draft or evaporation can lower her temperature dangerously. This is why babies should not be bathed in the first hour of life – this hot water and cold air destabilizes their temperature. If the baby gets cold, the surfactant in the lungs can stop working.

If a baby is separated from her mother her temperature changes chaotically. Temperature control uses calories which are the same calories which she should be using to grow. During protest she is using up these calories by crying and waving her arms and legs so there is less growth. During the despair stage she saves her calories to survive for longer. She does not release them for growing. Either way your baby will gain less weight. (It is hard to get enough food energy or calories into these tiny babies and they have so little fat reserves, so keeping their temperatures constant is one way of helping them save energy).

There are two technical words linked to temperature. **Hypothermia** means the body is too cold; **hyperthermia** means the body is too hot. A healthy temperature range is 96.5 to 99.5°F (36 to 37.5°C).

Incubators are used to keep premies warm. This is done in a variety of ways: with closed incubators, overhead heaters, infrared lights, open incubators and water beds.

> **The mother's chest regulates the baby's temperature better than any incubator ever can. Skin-to-Skin Contact keeps the temperature in the higher range and constant.**

Mom, with your naked baby skin-to-skin on your chest, your body will immediately warm by 3°F to warm your baby if it is cold; and your temperature can drop by 1°F to cool her if she is too warm. This is called "Thermal Synchrony".

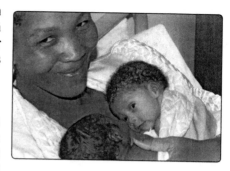

Research has shown that the mother's breasts act independently! If there are twins who have different temperatures, one breast cools, while the other warms. Aren't mothers' bodies amazing!

Your baby?		

Monitoring of the premature baby

Your baby has been born too early and is very fragile. The NICU staff will monitor your baby to make sure that there is progress, and to make sure that your baby is well and protected.

You may find your eyes fixed to the monitors, but remember that your own sense of your baby's well-being is the best monitor there is. You are her constant caregiver, while the nurses change in shifts and doctors come and go. She is your child and you will be the most sensitive to small changes in her condition. Look at her color; listen to her breathing, movements, awakeness, eye contact, restlessness and skin texture. Tell the nurse if you notice even a small change. You, Mom and Dad, can be the most sensitive monitors of your baby's progress.

> **Your own gut feeling of your baby's present condition is very likely to be correct!**

Continue to ask about the charts, and realize that there will be ups and downs. Also try to learn how to check if the monitors are properly attached. The graphs on the monitors will go up and down and show irregularities; this may be difficult for you emotionally. Try to look for the bigger trends, rather than the small ups and downs.

Labwork and other tests

Some of the basic tests are X-rays (XR) and ultrasounds (US). These tests assess baby's bones and basic organs. Blood tests check blood sugar levels, electrolytes and other chemicals in the blood. Bilirubin is one of the most commonly done tests. Bilirubin increases if the immature liver cannot remove the contents of broken down blood cells fast enough, this is called jaundice. If the bilirubin level is too high, it can damage the brain. If her bilirubin is raised, your baby will need to be under phototherapy lights, which help break down the bilirubin.

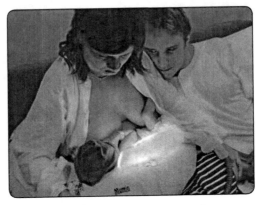

Baby in phototherapy on mother

Some tests on newborns are "<u>non-invasive</u>" like an ECG. These tests can be done when we need essential information and there is no risk for the child.

Other tests are "<u>minimally invasive</u>". Here the doctors and nurses have to balance the risk of not having information with the very small risk of harm while getting the information.

Other tests are "<u>invasive</u>". The risk for harm is high but the benefit is greater, they may be needed for survival, e.g., an arterial catheter.

As her parents, you should be consulted about all the tests your baby needs and be given time to ask questions about them, especially if you know the risk of harm is real. You need to give your consent – a signed consent form is needed in some hospitals.

Any painful procedure should have pain relief. Remember that Skin-to-Skin Contact and breastfeeding both relieve pain so you can use them together when painful procedures are performed on your baby. For example, a heel prick to collect blood may be needed: your baby needs your closeness to help her cope better.

Monitoring includes checking the various chemicals in your baby's blood. Some of these tests can be done with a small amount of blood from a heel prick; others will need more blood drawn from a vein, and blood gases are usually measured from an artery.

These are some of the tests that can be done on your baby in the NICU. The tests and their names vary between hospitals and countries. You could fill in your baby's tests below.

	Weight	usually done daily.
	Head circumference	weekly.
	Length	measured weekly in some hospitals, others do not see it as important at all.
Dx	Dextrose checks	these are done hourly for the first three hours, then 3 hourly for 24 hours to check blood sugar levels.
	Electrolytes	Sodium, potassium and other salts, checks kidney function also.
	Blood gases	these check oxygen and carbon dioxide in the blood. These are routine done if baby is on CPAP or a ventilator.
	Haematocrit	tests blood level; done at birth, then weekly.

BR	Bilirubin test	done if the baby is becoming jaundiced. Often done 6 hours after delivery and repeated after 12 hours.
CRP	C Reactive Protein	important if there is an infection.
LFT	Liver function test	done weekly if the staff are concerned about infection or if liver is enlarged.
CaPO4	Calcium phosphate	may be done if the baby does not grow in the first week and the staff suspect rickets.
FBC	Full blood count	done if infection is suspected, checks different things in blood.
	Urine test	screens for various changes in kidney function.
	Ultrasound of head	done if the head circumference increases and the staff suspect IVH (intraventricular hemorrhage).
CXR	Chest X Rays	shows lungs and heart
AXR	Abdominal X rays	shows stomach and intestines
US	Ultrasound	Shows different organs in body, also used in "echo" to look at heart working.
ECG	Electrocardiogram	measures the electrical activity in the heart.
Your Baby?		

Protection of the premature baby.

Monitoring usually includes protecting the physical needs of the body, but often neglects protecting the brain from stress. The baby also needs immunity which includes the antibodies in her blood and breastmilk which also provides her food. On top of all these is emotional security which is vital for all newborns and even more so for a fragile premature baby.

Most importantly, baby needs the immune protection provided by her mother's milk. More than 90% of the contents of human breastmilk are for protection.

Inside the mother the fetus is protected by the muscles of the uterus. Sounds are muted, it is dark and warm, and sensations are mostly calm and pleasurable. The baby is in a secure, fixed place, in close relationship to her mother.

Mother IS baby's protection.

More and more modern research is showing how the mother provides all the aspects of protection and that a baby needs continuity with her mother for healthy development.

> **If a baby is separated from her mother when she is born, she feels completely unprotected, vulnerable, alone, insecure and stressed.**
> **Technology may be needed to assist your baby to cope with the changes at birth, as an add-on, but not as a substitute for Mom.**
> **The preterm baby is even more dependent on her mother.**

The technology that has developed in the NICU often separates a premature baby from her mother. The lights may be too bright for her eyes, she has no way of closing her ears to all the many voices and beeping machine sounds in a busy NICU.

She needs protection against the pain of heel pricks, protection against over-stimulation and immunity against bacterial, viral and yeast infections. She needs protection against stress and the emotional trauma of separation for correct brain development. Her sensory needs are for "soft care" (see the section on developmental care).

> **You, Mom and Dad, are far superior for your baby than the incubator, in every way!**

Below is space to fill in any extra abbreviations below that are used in your NICU. Ask the staff to fill them in and explain them to you.

Again: DO NOT BE INTIMIDATED by the machinery.

Here are some practical things that you can do for your tiny baby as you sit with her for hours in the NICU, staring at the monitors or at her in an incubator.

- If an alarm goes off on your baby's machinery, it is for a reason. Do not ignore the alarm. You may need to go and call a nurse to ask why the alarm has gone off.

- Check the temperature controls of the incubator. If the temperature is above 99,5°F, you should alert a nurse.

- If your baby is having phototherapy for jaundice, always check that her eyes are properly covered with thick, dark cloth.

- The clip of the oxygen saturation probe with the red light needs to be moved every 3–6 hours, moving from left to right hand to right foot to left foot.

- Check that the intravenous line is flowing and the 'drip site' is not swollen and the skin around it is not red. Check that the fingers are not swelling. Sometimes there are small bubbles in the drip line, but there should not be big bubbles.

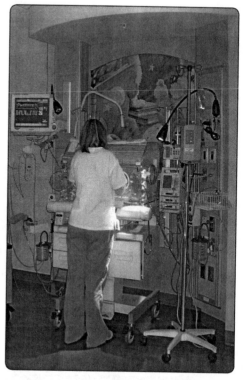

Often NICU babies need lots of machinery

Each hospital or NICU has different policies and routines and treatments and a professional team is there to help you and your baby to survive. Survival is the most urgent, important aspect for the NICU team – but increasingly we are aware that the quality of survival is important. This is your important work, Mom and Dad!

Appreciate the NICU team but realize that they cannot replace you as your baby's parent. You can and should politely insist on being there as much as possible.

Mom and Dad make the difference to the <u>quality</u> of survival.
This is measured in neurodevelopment.

The team can help your premie to survive physically, but to make the best of her fragile situation, she needs you.

<u>To encourage you, answer the following questions (use words or give a percentage).</u>

1. How much of this did you know before your baby was born? ....

2. How much of this did you know after one week? ....

3. How much of this do you know now ? ....

....

You have already learned a huge amount which will help you to cope so that you can help your baby in the best way possible!

Does your hospital or NICU

encourage you to be part of the caring team?...

allow you to be central to the caring team?...

answer your questions?..

explain what treatment they are giving and why? ....

<u>Please let us know how we can improve this information to help other parents.</u>

email to jill@kangaroomothercare.com
or write to: Jill Bergman, 8 Francis Road, Pinelands, 7405, Cape Town, South Africa

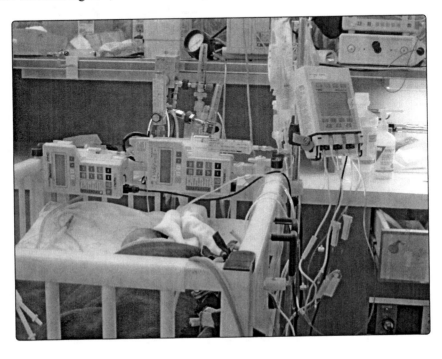

PROBLEMS PREMIES MAY FACE IN THE NICU

Entering the NICU and seeing all of the machines and tubes around tiny babies will probably feel really scary for you as parents. It will all be new and unfamiliar.

Try to ask questions of the staff and find out as much as you can about problems that your own baby may have. Some nurses don't want to give you too many details of what could go wrong as they don't want you to worry. Other staff members feel that it is best to tell parents everything so that they can cope and face the worst.

How much do YOU want to know: Mom ? ………   Dad? ……………

Ask the nurses to explain what is happening. Generally the more you know, the better you cope as parents of a premie and can help care for your baby. The more you understand, the more you can help. Try to trust. This is not to worry you, but to inform you.

> Firstly, do NOT presume that any or all of these apply to your baby!

There are many technical terms for the common problems of prematurity; this is a very simplified alphabetical list of the most common problems for everyday people to understand. Because the terms are so long, nurses and doctors often use abbreviations.

After the list you will see some of the longer-term problems premies may face as they grow.

This list is not for reading, it is for quick reference and is in alphabetical order. It is also for you to ask your doctor or nurse for details that apply to your baby and can be used for note-taking.

		Apnea	Pauses in breathing lasting more than 20 seconds. The baby "forgets" to breathe as her brain is immature. The heart rate slows and the baby becomes more "blue". She may need caffeine or theophylline to stimulate her and she often needs an apnea monitor She may need CPAP or medicine to help her breathe. This can be very scary for parents.
A's and B's		Apnea and Bradycardia	Apnea: lack of breathing (sometimes treated with caffeine). Bradycardia: very slow heart rate.
		Anemia	The baby may have too few red blood cells which carry oxygen to the body. She may need a blood transfusion.
		Asystole	The heart stops beating (but it will start again!).
BPD		Bronchopulmonary dysplasia	The lungs of a premie are immature, and are at risk of developing abnormally with inflammation and scarring, long term oxygen support may be needed.
		Cardiac arrest	The heart stops beating (but it will start again!).

CP	Cerebral Palsy	There is damage to the brain before or during birth. There can be weakness of arms, legs or face, but this is often not seen until later in life.
	Collapsed lung	This is caused by a hole in a lung. It may need an "underwater drain" into the chest cage which bubbles under water to open the lung.
GER	Gastro-esophageal reflux	This is vomiting up food (called "spitting up" in the USA). Reflux can also be acidic food in the esophagus that causes pain.
	Hydrocephalus	This translates as "water in the head". It is actually spinal fluid in the ventricles of the brain. The baby's head may swell and there is increased pressure on the brain. The baby may need a shunt to get rid of the extra fluid.
	Hyperbilirubinemia	See jaundice
	Hyperglycemia	This is difficulty with sugar balance: premie babies sometimes have blood sugar levels that are too high.
	Hypoglycemia	Premies far more commonly have blood sugar levels that are too low.
IVH	Intraventricular hemorrhage	This is bleeding inside the ventricles, which are fluid filled chambers in the middle of the brain. Small bleeds are common and clear up, large ones may cause problems.
	Jaundice or hyperbilirubinemia	The baby's skin becomes yellow, old red blood cells are broken down in the liver and the body cannot get rid of bilirubin, the waste product. She may need phototherapy under ultraviolet lights.
NEC	Necrotizing enterocolitis	Premie babies have immature intestines and sometimes an infection can cause part of the intestines to die. This is very serious, and should be treated early before there is damage.
PDA	Patent ductus arteriosus	Before birth, the PDA lets blood flow directly to the fetus' body instead of to the lungs. The duct that allows this normally closes at birth; in a premie this may not have closed yet.
	Pneumonia	Lung infection
	Pneumothorax	This is caused by a hole in a lung, which collapses it partially or completely, she may need an "underwater drain" into the chest cage which bubbles under water to open the lung.
PPHN	Persistent pulmonary hypertension	Blood vessels to and around the lungs are small and tight. They should be relaxed and open so the baby can get enough oxygen.

PVL	Periventricular leukomalacia	This refers to damage to brain tissue caused by decreased blood flow.
RDS	Respiratory distress syndrome	A premie baby's lungs are immature and cannot produce surfactant. The baby may breathe too fast or "grunt". She may need extra oxygen by CPAP or breathing machine, a ventilator or respirator.
ROP	Retinopathy of prematurity	Premies' eyes are sensitive to too much oxygen, and blood vessels can grow abnormally in the retina.
	Seizures	Another name for fitting, can be caused by low blood sugar, mineral imbalance, infections or brain bleeds.
	Sepsis	Infection generally, but often refers to infection in blood stream.
SIDS	Sudden Infant Death Syndrome	This can affect any baby, but premies are more likely to have SIDS. Breastfeeding, lying the baby on her back, safe sleeping and NO SMOKING for parents of premies can help prevent SIDS.
TTN	Transient Tachypnea of the Newborn	Also called "wet lungs", baby breathes too fast because of extra fluid not being cleared out of lungs in the first hours of life.
Your Baby?		

LONG TERM PROBLEMS PREMIES MAY FACE & HOW SKIN-TO-SKIN CONTACT CAN HELP

Modern medical science has advanced so much that far more very tiny babies of 26 or even 22 weeks gestation are surviving. There are still questions as to the QUALITY of that survival and how many problems this tiny baby and her parents will have to cope with as she grows (1).

Premies have not had an ideal start as they were born too early. It is known that babies born premature have in the past had less developed brains than full term babies. **Now we believe that this need not be so.** Even extremely premature babies can do very well.

If a baby is born before 26 weeks there is a high risk of major developmental problems which may cause difficulties or delays later on. Under 24 or 25 weeks of gestation the number of problems premies face is very much greater (2).

> "I would hope that people understand that being born early is a very, very serious business, that survival is not high, and that should children survive, their likelihood of having life-long problems – particularly in respect of learning – is high".
>
> **"We need to do all that we can to find ways to bridge the baby's developmental gap and to nurture healthy brain development outside the womb."**
>
> – *Professor Kate Costeloe* (3)

Holding your baby in Skin-to-Skin Contact can help bridge this gap.

You as a parent will want to do all you can to minimize these problems. In the past premies have had a one in ten risk of cerebral palsy, a quarter may need help at school and have lower IQ. Forty percent of survivors have moderate to severe problems in brain development. Interestingly, boys are twice as likely to have problems later than girls (2).

This list is not to scare or depress you and none of it may apply to your baby, but if your expectations are realistic it is sometimes easier to cope. Facing the issues and having information about them may help you to cope better. Even more importantly, it will help show you how important it is that you are with your tiny baby holding her skin-to-skin to help her development to prevent problems later on. This is how this workbook began: "If only I had known, I would have done things differently..."

A common question is, "What can I expect in terms of development?"

Let's look at mental, physical and emotional development for babies separated from parents compared to those in Skin-to-Skin Contact.

Mental Development

<u>Separated premies</u> are at greater risk of

    brain bleeds (IVH) from stress and separation from their mothers;

    less brain development (1;4) and

    fewer neural pathways.

They are also at greater risk of developing learning and attention problems like ADD, ADHD (5;6) and possibly autism spectrum disorder (ASD).

Skin-to-skin contact can help protect your baby. In the first days after birth, your baby held in Skin-to-Skin Contact is calm and unstressed, and her brain is being wired for health. Also she does not cry, and therefore is less likely to have a brain bleed.

Developmentally, Skin-to-Skin Contact is important over the first months for the "approach" brain pathways. Being with your baby will protect her sleep for healthy brain wiring; protect her eyes from bright lights; her ears from loud sounds; her nose from strong smells and her skin from rough handling and pain. All of these will protect her brain from the bad effects of stress.

Physical Development

Separated premies are at greater risk of

> cerebral palsy,
>
> delayed motor development,
>
> delayed speech development,
>
> feeding problems,
>
> blindness, or
>
> deafness (1).

If a premie lies on her back in an incubator for a month or two with her legs flopped out sideways, her hips may be rotated outwards, which could make crawling, and later walking, more difficult. Such a premie will walk with her toes turned outward. This could cause her to be teased, which further lowered her self-esteem in later years. Her motor skills of smiling, sitting, crawling, walking, speaking may well be delayed because of low muscle tone.

If she lies on her back in an incubator, her chest muscles can stretch and her back muscles shrink, and she may not even be able to get her arms to midline. This can make it harder for her to push herself up from her tummy and learn to crawl later. Delaying crawling can delay her speech development and mathematics ability. Often nothing is done until the child reaches preschool age. Start supporting her development in the NICU and you will have far fewer problems later.

Lying on her back can make her head flatter.

Skin-to-skin contact can help protect your baby in the first days after birth. She will not be as stressed so her heart rate, blood pressure and breathing and temperature will stay more constant. She will start breastfeeding earlier, absorb her food better and so grow faster. Holding her upright and flexed on your chest helps the spine to learn to balance and increases muscle tone. If she is in an incubator, positioning her comfortably can make a huge difference.

Skin-to-Skin Contact and breastfeeding go together so here is a small note about the long-term benefits of breastfeeding. The action of suckling from the breast is needed to strengthen her jaw muscles and shape her jaw and mouth for later speech development and straight teeth. The American Academy of Pediatrics recommends that mothers exclusively breastfeed their infants up to six months of age (7), and that nursing for a year or more will give a baby the "full benefits of breastfeeding," which include cutting rates of illnesses such as ear infections and diarrhea and reducing the risk of childhood obesity. Babies should be breastfed for 2 years to grow to their maximum brain growth.

Emotional Development

Separated premies have spent a lot of time alone in an incubator in NICU, and so are stressed and dissociate emotionally. They may not bond or make good attachment to their parents or to others very easily. This can cause them huge problems emotionally and socially throughout their lives.

Skin-to-skin contact can help your baby as she will feel emotionally safe, calm and loved. You provide your baby with the only familiar constant to give her emotional security, and help her catch up on what she has missed. On your chest your premie can reach stability more easily (self-regulate). By putting her in the fetal position with her arms close to her chest and near her mouth you will help your premie to self-comfort and stabilize her body and her emotions. Your voice talking and singing to her will be reassuring.

Mom and Dad, your baby will trust you and feel safe with you and bond with you, and so be secure enough to bond with an increasing number of people, starting with family and friends. This will help her to build healthy relationships and will encourage long-term benefits throughout her life.

Skin-to-Skin Contact between a baby and adoptive parents can have a hugely positive impact on bonding and building trust.

These simple things can have a profound impact on minimizing problems later on. If this means taking time off work for a few weeks to be in the NICU with your baby, do it. It can save you many months or years of problems later. It is a very worthwhile investment of time! If parents have to work, having one constant care-giver can provide a good base for development.

Some studies have even suggested that working parents can give a child the basic bonding time that she needs for healthy development by allowing her to co-sleep with them.

> **There are many things that your premie can catch up over the first few years. Early professional help can make a huge difference to your baby's outcome. Get a physiotherapist involved AS EARLY AS POSSIBLE. He or she can draw up a set of exercises and activities for you to work on with your baby as early as you can. This can start with infant massage, and go on to tiny exercises in the NICU. The first few weeks and months of a baby's life are crucial.**

Get help early

Remember that the baby has the most brain cells or neurons at 28 weeks gestation. These neurons are branching and connecting at synapses and are busiest in the first year of life. The "metabolic activity" in the brain is highest until 3 years of life; after this it slows down. Focus on supporting your baby in these first three years. Do not wait to discover problems at preschool; it will be very much more difficult then.

Some say that premies are behind and will "catch up" to their normal developmental milestones by two or three years. Others say that premies never fully catch up. The truth is somewhere in between, and will often depend on the individual baby. Expect delays!

It may feel like there is a long road ahead of you: ask for help from family and friends and health professionals; get advice; join with other parents of premies, read about prematurity; BE there for your baby. She needs your love; she needs you to be her champion. Work together and keep talking as a couple or family. Your premie needs as much help as she can get to make up for her early start. Most of all, she needs YOU, her parents, close to her, and your love can help to pull her through this rough start to life.

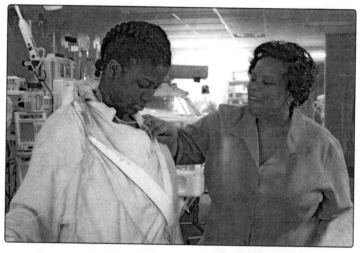

Ask for help from family and friends.

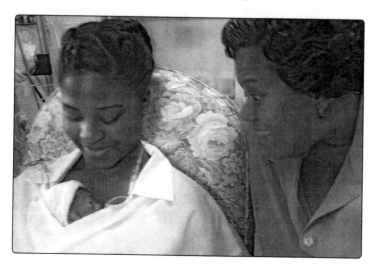

Fine Print Page – Long term problems premies may face

1. This articles reviews cerebral palsy primarily, and then more broadly developmental outcomes from very low birth weight babies. "VLBW infants remain at substantial risk for a wide spectrum of long-term morbidity including cerebral palsy (CP), mental retardation, developmental delay, school problems, behavioral issues, growth failure, and overall poor health status."
2. The smaller the babies, (<1000g) the worse the long term outcomes, but not always!
3. The EPICURE study from the UK is one of the most rigorous, with long term follow-up data.
4. An MRI study of brains of preterm infants, showing that they have not grown as they would have in the uterus.
5. ADD and ADHD are approximately 3 times more common in premies.
6. Cognitive impairment is also related to decreasing gestational age at birth.
7. Breastfeeding and breastmilk are protective.

Reference List

(1) Wilson-Costello D. Is there evidence that long-term outcomes have improved with intensive care? Seminars In Fetal & Neonatal Medicine 2007 October 16;12(5):344-54.

(2) Vohr BR, Wright LL, Dusick AM, Mele L, Verter J, Steichen JJ et al. Neurodevelopmental and functional outcomes of extremely low birth weight infants in the National Institute of Child Health and Human Devel-opment Neonatal Research Network, 1993-1994. Pediatrics 2000 June;105(6):1216-26.

(3) Costeloe K, Wood NS Gibson AT, Hennessy EM, Marlow N, Wilkinson AR. The EPICure study: associa-tions and antecedents of neurological and developmental disability at 30 months of age following extremely preterm birth. Archives of Disease in Childhood -- Fetal & Neonatal Edition 2005 March;90(2):F134-F140.

(4) Inder TE, Warfield SK, Wang H, Huppi PS, Volpe JJ. Abnormal cerebral structure is present at term in pre-mature infants. Pediatr 2005;115(2):286-94.

(5) Botting N, Powls A, Cooke RWI. Attention deficit hyperactivity disorders and other psychiatric outcomes in very low birth weight children at 12 years. J Child Psychol Psychiatry 1997;38(8):931-41.

(6) Cooke RW, Foulder-Hughes L. Growth impairment in the very preterm and cognitive and motor perform-ance at 7 years. Arch Dis Child 2003;88(6):482-7.

(7) American Academy of Pediatric : Section on Breastfeeding. Breastfeeding and the use of human milk. Ameri-can Academy of Pediatrics 2005;115(2):496-506.

HOW FRIENDS AND FAMILY CAN HELP

The birth of a child should be a wonderful experience in any family. The birth of a premature baby can be very difficult and brings its own mixture of joy, sadness and worry.

Parents, do ask for help!!

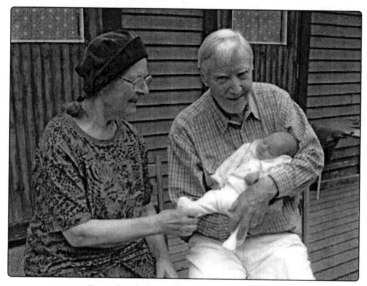

Grandparents can be a huge support.

Ask your family and friends to support you in whatever ways they can. They can help by <u>not</u> coming in to the NICU as this will be stressful for your baby and other babies there and bring in unnecessary germs.

Friends and family can have a huge role to play in supporting the parents of a premature infant.

It is often difficult to repeat all the news of your baby. Give details of your premie's progress to one family member or friend. Everyone else can contact them and not disturb you. This can reduce your stress. Maybe you could get that person to send out a weekly email with a photo. Some parents keep friends updated with "facebook" etc.

Parents, do not try to be strong and cope on your own.

There are people who want to and can help you.

There is little that friends and family can do to help the premie baby directly, but here are some practical ideas from parents of premies themselves of what they would like help with!

Some things to do

Offer practical support, e.g. being with the older siblings of the premie while mom and dad to go to the hospital.

Grannies, aunts and friends can be a huge help by being stand-in caregivers for older siblings at home.

Let the parents talk freely.

Offer to do washing.

Offer to take the siblings to school.

Give support.

Phone and ask how you can help or send a text message on a mobile phone. Parents can read this when it suits them. Don't expect an answer!

Email your support.

Offer to hold the baby while mom sleeps when she gets home. She will often feel too tired to "entertain you".

Cook meals and answer phones, especially when the premie baby gets home.

Offer to go shopping.

Later, baby-sit when the premie is bigger – encourage Mom and Dad to go out for coffee together.

Some things to avoid

Do not all go and visit the NICU – that takes too many foreign germs into the hospital and will stress the tiny baby.

Don't ask if the baby will survive – the parents and doctors do not know and it is a huge worry for them.

Don't ask lots of questions.

Don't give lots of "advice".

Do not take photographs with a flash as it will hurt the premie's eyes.

Do not ask how long she will be in NICU – the parents and nurses do not know.

Do not blame the parents as if it was their "fault" that they had a premie.

Don't tell parents to "be strong" or "forget your baby for now and come out with us".

Do not pretend that the baby does not exist, especially if she died. The premie was a very real person for that mother and father and always will be. Do not say, "you can always have another baby."

Don't visit the parents when you are sick.

Do not visit in the first weeks after the premie gets home. Let the family settle down at home first. Be sensitive to their needs.

Do not be offended if the parents will not let you hold their premie baby. They have fought for her life and she feels more secure with them.

Do not _ever_ smoke in the same room as a premie. It can increase her risk of SIDS and she will be much more likely to get infections.

Do not take offence if parents of premies seem irritable or angry with you. They are coping with an extremely stressful situation and need your support.

GOING HOME

When can my baby go home or be "discharged"?

This is very individual and depends on how early your premie was born, if she needed oxygen or surgery. Different hospitals have different measures or criteria for when a premie is ready to go home, for example when she is a certain weight or gestational age.

You can go home when

- you, the parents feel confident to care for your premie baby alone;
- your baby is exclusively breastfeeding, or she is feeding properly from breast or a cup;
- she is gaining weight continuously;
- she can keep her own body temperature normal;
- her heart and lungs are working properly;
- home is safe and mother has support and follow-up care.

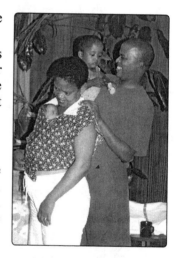

Ideally, parents should have already been doing all the care in the NICU for some time.

Many hospitals have a "rooming in" time for 24 hours for parents to learn all the care of their premie. Do ask for this so that you can care for all of the needs of your premie while you still have the support of the NICU staff, so that you can gain confidence.

Important

Your tiny baby is still premature and should not be left alone at home. She will still need very "intensive care" but from you, not from machines. Carrying your baby skin-to-skin in a KangaCarrier or sling will help you to continue to give your baby the best care while doing your home chores.

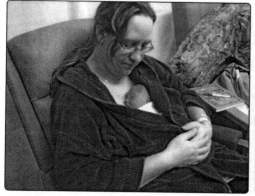

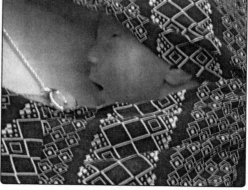

Going home may bring up a mixture of feelings in you. It is an exciting but sometimes scary time. You might feel relieved that you're home and not having to go to the hospital every day. Sometimes your premie has been in the NICU for many weeks, so it is a huge adjustment for you as parents to be completely responsible for her full time care, 24 hours a day. You may feel tired as there are no nurses to be care-givers while you take a break. Your premie baby may need to feed 10–14 times a day!

You may feel anxious that there are no nurses to support you or even monitors, and you may be worried that you may not be able to cope.

You may find yourself always worrying about your baby and often checking that she is breathing properly. You can sometimes feel lonely or isolated now that you are alone at home after the busy NICU. All of these are normal reactions! Be kind to yourself!

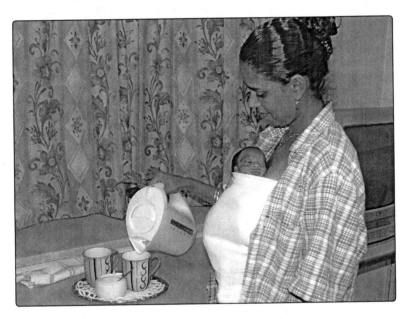

Going home checklists

Do you know how to

- give your baby all the care she needs;
- feed her as often as possible;
- change her nappy or diaper;
- calm your baby;
- give her a bath;
- give her medicines;
- put her safely in car seat (premies are too small for normal car seats – roll towels at the sides);
- do baby CPR;
- use the equipment;
- work the apnea monitor if she needs oxygen?

Do you know

if all your baby's immunizations and tests have been done;

who her doctor will be;

what immunizations she needs;

know if/when tests need to be done, e.g., eye, hearing, ultrasound?

Do you have

support at home

safety numbers – Doctor, NICU, Lactation Consultants, social workers, clinics,

all the premie clothes that you need (they need to be SOFT inside for her delicate skin);

premie diapers/nappies (as small as possible);

a breast pump if you need it;

a discharge summary from the hospital of your baby's treatments, etc;

a list of follow-up appointments at the clinic and for the 18 week corrected age check up;

all her medicines if she needs any?

Some ideas for when you get home

Rest at home.

Make time to bond with your baby.

Try to make home peaceful.

Make your premie's "playtime" with siblings short – she needs to rest and sleep to grow.

Keep the home temperature constant.

If your premie is sweating, take off her clothes.

You and the family should wash your hands often. Visitors especially need to wash their hands.

Get a phone answering machine.

No "pass the parcel" with visitors – keep your premie skin-to-skin on your chest.

Your ideas (your discharge nurse can help you here):

....

....

....

....

....

....

....

> ### The best advice I got when I had a newborn baby was:
>
> ### SLEEP WHEN SHE SLEEPS!

As you leave the hospital with your premie, here are some things which <u>developmental follow-ups will need to include</u>:

>   regular weight checks;
>
>   head circumference measurements;
>
>   a developmental assessment every six months;
>
>   regular hearing and eye examinations;
>
>   check-ups with a speech therapist.

Your premie may need some physiotherapy help, especially in the first three years.

Some countries have "early intervention programs" to follow up babies that have been born prematurely. Join these if you can.

<u>Things to be aware of</u>.

>   Does your baby turn her head towards light and sound?
>
>   Does your baby move her head if you hold a bright object and move it from side to side?
>
>   Does she reach for things with both hands?

Ask your doctor or physiotherapist for daily exercises to do with your premie to strengthen her muscles and help her to develop "normally". Remember that the more little things you do early in her life, the more impact they will have. Do spend this time helping your baby, especially in the first few months and years. It will be the best investment of time that you could ever make.

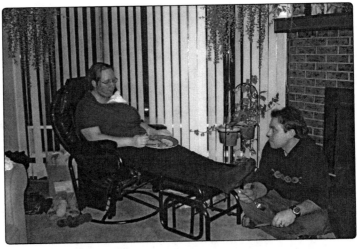

Baby in SSC as mom and dad are at home.

PARENTING

This chapter applies for every baby, but even more so for a sensitive baby. Premies are more likely to be sensitive.

There are many good books on parenting in the resources section, but you may not have time to read them now. Some books may be out of date and give advice which will not work for your baby.

Based on science, here are some important things to do (1). A lot of this is also "common sense", but some of these things seem to have been forgotten in western society and lost in technology.

<u>Trust your instincts! (2)</u>

If your baby cries, your natural reaction will be to pick her up and comfort her. This is the right reaction, so ignore the books that say "train her to sleep by leaving her to cry". There is no science to support their arguments.

<u>Breastfeed</u>:

Parents who carry their babies in Skin-to-Skin Contact are more likely to breastfeed their babies and breastfeed for much longer with all the huge benefits (3). The American Academy of Pediatrics recommends breastfeeding for two years (4). The Skin-to-Skin Contact stimulates the release of prolactin and oxytocin hormones which help in breastmilk production.

<u>Bonding</u>:

Babies need to belong! If mom and baby have bonded well in the first hours and days and weeks of life, this will make it easier for your baby to trust and bond with others. "Attachment parenting" works because of basic biology, which happens because of Skin-to-Skin Contact (1;5). Your baby on your chest at birth starts the hormones in you and your baby working together in the right way. This makes good parenting so much easier. You respond to your baby and give her what she needs.

When your baby is in the right place on your chest, she will have the "right" behavior of stable heart rate and breathing, breastfeeding, sleeping and waking in a regular rhythm, absorbing food maximally, and bonding with you. Human babies are born with a strong urge to self-regulate. If she is born prematurely, your baby will need your help to regulate, and your body can automatically calm her. Babies are also born with a deep inner drive to bond, belong and communicate with mom. Skin-to-Skin Contact helps these natural drives (as well as mothers' natural instinct to protect and provide for her baby).

Some parents may be reading this book and feel guilty that they did not give their premie early Skin-to-Skin Contact. You may have been in a NICU that did not understand the importance of this early bonding time. It is never too late to make contact with your baby or child. In adoption, Skin-to-Skin Contact will help with bonding. Lots of love and hugs, eye contact, focused listening to them and playing with them on their level can make your child feel more secure. Sitting reading to a bigger child with your arm around her will make a difference to her self-esteem.

Holding and carrying and "baby wearing":

Holding and carrying your baby skin-to-skin will allow your newborn to experience the outside world from a safe place (6). Babies like to feel contained and be held quiet and still. This helps bonding and also encourages the mother to carry and hold her child for the first two years of life. This is what babies need for best brain-wiring and emotional security. This is particularly important during the first six to eight weeks for the part of the brain called the amygdala, which controls emotions. Carrying the baby is still very important after eight weeks. If you have twins, Dad, Granny or an aunt can carry a twin skin-to-skin. However, for the best effects for breastfeeding it would need to be mother, so each twin has a turn on mom.

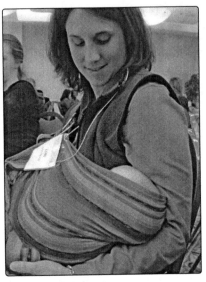

Babies love to be carried. Hold and carry for the first 2 years.

Carrying the full term baby skin-to-skin can be done with any sling. When carrying a premature baby it is essential to stabilize the baby's airway. A KangaCarrier® will do this (see page 49).

Swaddling and loud noise ("shushing") may get a baby to "settle". While this looks like sleep, the baby's brain may be in "freeze", a defense reflex caused by threat. If this was so, it would be wiring stress and avoidance pathways in her brain (see page 88).

Talk with your baby:

Talk to your baby to help make the best brain connections. It is worth investing time looking at your baby, playing with her and making eye-to-eye contact (1). It is important for Dad to spend time doing this too. Be sensitive to avoid over-whelming her. Remember that your premie may easily be over-stimulated and so start to focus elsewhere. Respect that and give her a break.

Reading to your baby and young child has huge benefits. Singing and playing music has an organizing effect on brain function.

Get involved:

Guard your baby's sense of security. Be careful not to let your newborn tiny baby be held by too many

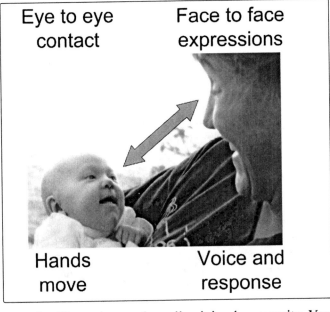

Eye to eye contact

Face to face expressions

Hands move

Voice and response

people. She feels safest with your familiar voices and smells giving her security. You also want to reduce the risk of infections.

If your baby's crying is prolonged when she is left at crèche or day care centre, consider investing time in your child's long term security by being at home with her for a while longer. Work will still be there in several months! It is the best investment of time you will ever make in your life! "Being there" applies for toddlers as well. If they are held close, then allowed to explore to someone else, and return to check that mom is still there, then go out again, they will be much more trusting, secure and confident.

> ### BE there for your child.

BEING there for your children is important for all ages. (It still applies when they are teenagers!) Being there means your interested and active involvement as well as time and love.

Time and love:

Babies spell LOVE as T-I-M-E.

You cannot "spoil" a baby till 2–3 years. You cannot "over-love" a baby. But you can certainly "damage" a baby by loving it too little (7)!

Babies do take time! There are no short-cuts to love. In our fast-paced society, slowing down to BE present with your baby, will help your baby and will help you set more balanced priorities in your own life. Your baby is an individual person and needs to be respected as such, and talked to and listened to. Do fill up your baby's emotional tank by allowing her "cuddle time" and nurture her properly. The benefits will last a lifetime! Play with your baby as she grows. Play brings together all of the touch, eye contact, laughter and movement that are essential for brain wiring. In neuroscience, play is building the circuits to prepare for adult life.

Sleeping:

Many books on baby care offer parents advice on "sleep training" to get their baby to sleep through the night. While this is convenient and desirable for you as parents, research shows that babies do not sleep through the night. They wake, but keep quiet because they have learnt that no one will comfort them and provide their basic biological needs for food or for love, or warmth or security.

> **"Controlled crying" is a very harsh infant sleep training technique and should not be used with young babies (if at all with any children!).**
> *– Professor H.L. Ball*

Co-sleeping:

The debates around co-sleeping are endless. Parents and babies sometimes struggle to coordinate their times of sleeping, so parents often get very tired! As this book is based on the biology of mother-baby Skin-to-Skin Contact, I will be using the term co-sleeping to mean sleeping in the same bed. A side cot that allows your arm to sense your baby's waking movements also works well. Sleep with a firm flat mattress with your arm close to your baby. Sleeping in this way allows your baby to breastfeed without waking you! You will both sleep better and so enjoy those early months far more!

The biological fact remains that babies benefit enormously from that close physical contact with Mom. Your arm close to your baby can sense her needs and distress signals quickly. For this to work, just sleeping in the same room is not enough. Sleep cycling is critical for brain wiring, and good sleep cycling only takes place in mother's presence. Babies in Skin-to-Skin Contact do not sink into deep sleep in which they stop breathing (apnea, which may lead to SIDS or cot death).

But just as we drive a car safely with seat belts and with babies in special baby seats, so co-sleeping must be done SAFELY. I will speak strongly here for your baby's safety! Moms and dads who smoke and co-sleep with their baby increase her risk of SIDS, so parents should not smoke, nor take drugs. This also means for you to keep your baby sleeping safely in your bed, you should not drink alcohol. Do not have loose duvets or big pillows. Sleeping with baby in a sofa or armchair is dangerous.

It has been suggested that working parents who have their babies in a daycare can have their babies sleeping in their beds and this makes a difference to their baby's emotional stability.

Nurture different intelligences

We have written this book specifically about protecting and stimulating your own baby's brain. Each sensation has its own intelligence or wiring (9). Please remember there are lots of different ways in which people are "intelligent" or gifted.

Take time to watch your child as she plays and grows. Your role as a parent is to nurture your child, to learn and boost what your baby and later child is good at to build her self-esteem. Encourage her with things that she struggles with.

Some children are gifted at sport and dancing and learn best when they are moving. Other children are good with understanding three dimensions and are good with blocks and puzzles, and are artistic. Others are good with words. They like reading and writing and poems and other languages. They learn best by seeing things. Some children are very good with Math and enjoy the logic of chess, numbers and computers. Musicians enjoy sounds and rhythms and learn best by hearing things. Some children learn best working with others in a group as they are so good with people, while others prefer to be alone. Being outdoors and with animals is the best place for some children to learn.

Every child is different, unique and special and needs your encouragement to be that. Premies are sometimes delayed in some areas, so find those that she is good at. Encouraging all parts of her will help her grow up well-rounded and to reach her full potential as an individual.

Parenting twins and multiples

Twins and triplets have a higher risk of being born early so premies can also be multiples! That makes the first weeks and months at home even more of a challenge! Mothers of twins often say that you should wake the other twin when the first twin wakes, to try to get them feeding at the same time to protect your sleep (10;11).

If your twins are premature, place them together in an incubator for comfort facing each other. Better still place them together on your chest in Skin-to-Skin Contact.

Ask for help from family and friends! Be aware that caring for twins can also be an added stress on your relationship.

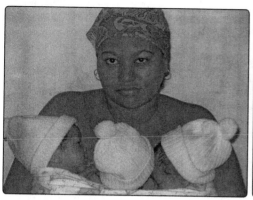 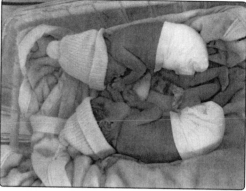

Notes/journaling space:

....

....

....

....

....

....

....

....

....

....

....

....

....

....

....

....

....

....

Parenting specifically for premies

This whole book has been about this topic!!

To summarize:

<u>For the first few weeks,</u> Skin-to-Skin Contact, mother's presence, breastfeeding, containment and a quiet environment are very helpful. Baby should be kept in flexion (legs and arms bent). Protect her sleep. Infant massage can be helpful. Do not leave her to cry.

<u>In the first months,</u>

Continue as above. Hold your baby and hug her lots. If you are reading this when your premie has grown a bit, it is never too late to give them extra hugs! Carry her as much a possible; she will sleep best this way! She will feel safe, and this will help her catch up her development.

Protect her sleep and do not wake her unnecessarily. Play with her when she is awake and start reading stories and singing songs.

Watch your baby to see how much stimulation she can cope with. Try not to overwhelm her. Start with small doses of stimulation and read her signals. Be sensitive to her. Hold a bright object above your baby's face. Move it from side to side to see if her eyes will follow it.

It is important for your baby to crawl, so from about three months of age put her down to lie on her tummy on the floor when she is awake for playing. She will start to lift her head and try to push herself up. This will strengthen upper body muscle tone. When she is sleeping, she can be on her back or side.

Avoid using a baby walker or walking ring for your baby. They do not help upper body tone and balance and they force her legs to move at an unnatural angle. The best is to carry your baby is a safe sling.

<u>Here are some practical things for you as a parent to do, or look out for.</u>

Check that your premie responds to sounds; if a door slams by mistake and she does not react at all, it may be worth checking her hearing.

Is your baby's body floppy if you hold her hands and pull her from lying to sitting position? When she is six months, can she sit? Does she usually fall over to the same side?

Encourage her to use both arms and both legs equally. Try to keep her supple by gentle exercises like bicycling with her legs and arms as you play with her.

Remember that she will need a lot of sleep and quiet play.

It is important to have regular checkups. These will assess for possible problems early on, when they are much easier to work on. Follow the advice your hospital gives you. If you are worried about anything, ask at your regular checkups. Premies have a lot to catch up and it may take time to do this. Be gentle with them; be grateful and celebrate small progress.

Do NOT expect them to do all the things at the same age as a full term baby can.

Fine Print Page – Parenting

1. This excellent Dorling Kindersley book covers parenting from birth to teenage years.
2. This short book summarizes evidence on the key role mothers play in child development. The book can be downloaded free from the internet, link at bottom of page, http://www.imhaanz.org.nz/peter-cooks-mothering-denied-available-internet.
3. Biological Nurturing is based on the same neuroscience described in this book. Skin-to-Skin Contact and breast-feeding impact all aspects of good development. http://www.biologicalnurturing.com/
4. Given the conservative medical culture of the USA, the recommendation of the AAP reflects the strength of the evidence now available.
5. This article from Mothering" magazine may be easier to read than some of the scientific references here.
6. Book now available from http://www.hale-publishing.com/
7. A practical and helpful little book.
8. Co-sleeping is controversial, and McKenna explains the issues in a way that is based on a broader and better understanding of the science. See website: http://www.nd.edu/~jmckenn1/lab/ Article can be downloaded from http://www.naturalchild.org/james_mckenna/cosleeping.pdf
9. Book may be challenging reading, but there are succinct summaries available on internet: http://www.davesab-ine.com/Music/Articles/MITheoryHowardGardner/tabid/170/Default.aspx
10–11. … two good books on managing twins at home!

Reference List

(1) Sunderland M. The Science of Parenting. Dorling Kindersley Limited, London; 2006.
(2) Cook P. Mothering denied. 2008.
(3) Colson S. Biological nurturing. Biological Nurturing 2005.
(4) American Academy of Pediatric : Section on Breastfeeding. Breastfeeding and the use of human milk. Ameri-can Academy of Pediatrics 2005;115(2):496-506.
(5) Porter LL. The science of attachment: The biological roots of love. Mothering 2003 July;(119).
(6) Blois M. Babywearing. Pharmasoft Publishing, L.P.; 2005.
(7) Contey C, Takikawa D. CALMS A guide to soothing your baby. Hana Peace Works, Los Olivos; 2007.
(8) McKenna JJ, McDade T. Why babies should never sleep alone. A review of the co-sleeping controversy in rela-tion to SIDS, bedsharing and breastfeeding. Paediatric Respiratory reviews 2005;6:134-1.
(9) Gardner HE. Frames of Mind: The Theory of Multiple Intelligences. New York: Basic Books; 1983.
(10) Gromada KK. Mothering Multiples. Third ed. , USA: La Leche League International; 1999.
(11) Noble E. Having Twins - and more. Houghton Mifflin Company; 2003.

COMPASSIONATE CARE FOR A DYING BABY

This is a really hard section and my heart goes out to parents in this situation.

Many people avoid talking about death, but it is important.

A baby represents new life and a future, the opposite of death. To watch a baby die does not follow the natural order of life.

If your baby is dying:

Many parents have been allowed to do skin-to-skin contact with their tiny baby even if she is dying. This is called compassionate care. (1). These parents have hugely valued being able to hold their tiny baby for the short time that they had together.

Adults do not want to die alone.
Do not leave your tiny baby to die alone.

Sometimes death occurs after weeks of struggling. Hold your baby as she dies. Give her permission to let go and stop struggling.

Give her a name; she is a real person and already has her own personality. It will help you to grieve her death appropriately.

If your baby has already died you may want to hold her to say goodbye. This can be important for you. Be aware that she may have a different skin color and be cold.

Collect mementos such as a lock of hair and her tiny armband from the hospital.

Take photos of her; this will help you to treasure the memory of your very real baby.

If your tiny premie dies it may be an intense shock for you and you may have extremely strong reactions of grief. All of these are normal reactions, so don't fear that you are going crazy. Your feelings may include sadness, anger, guilt, anxiety, helplessness, fatigue and relief. You may be physically numb, have tightness in your throat, lack energy, feel weak and be over-sensitive to noise. You may not believe that your baby has died or be confused. You may want to withdraw, lose your appetite, struggle to sleep, dream of your baby, sigh, cry and feel restless.

- Do have a proper funeral – this allows you to mourn and grieve properly, and friends and family will support you.
- Don't try to pretend your baby did not exist (2).
- Get help from professionals / support groups (3).
- Be aware of the risk of depression.

You may find yourself "searching", yearning for your lost one (3;4). You cannot forget your baby or replace her. You may grieve for different lengths of time from your partner; you may feel anger and want to blame someone.

Feelings of wanting to get back into normal life and reinvesting in life are sometimes very slow to return and may take months. Allow this time of grieving and emotional ups and downs or waves.

It is important to be very careful how you tell young siblings about death. Siblings may have had to cope with Mom being away in hospital for weeks with the premie baby and may feel very rejected and jealous of the baby who was getting all the attention. If the baby dies, they may blame themselves because they were feeling jealous of the baby.

Do be aware that if you have another pregnancy later, you may find yourself very anxious that this baby too may not survive. This is often overlooked. (4;5). Friends, family and medical staff will need to be extra supportive.

If you have a faith community or church, let the members support you. Be gentle with yourself. You have had a major life shock.

Fine Print Page – Compassionate Care

1. This is one of the earliest recorded cases, and the skin-to-skin contact was an important aspect. The parents were obviously also supported in many other ways.
2. Staff often find it difficult – even after training – to talk to bereaved parents. These authors … "offer this column as a vehicle for reflecting on the meanings of words used during this particular time of loss and grief."
3. This review article describes 19 publications on perinatal bereavement or distressing birth experience counseling, Quote: 'Counseling strategies provided women with opportunities to talk about their birth experience, express feelings about what happened, have questions answered, address gaps in knowledge or understanding of events, connect the event with emotions and behavior, talk about future pregnancies, and explore existen-tial issues." Conclusions about how effective these are cannot be drawn …, but that it is important is not questioned !!
4. A "Perinatal Bereavement Scale" is described, and it showed that "parents who have experienced a late peri-natal loss (stillbirth or neonatal death) display more unresolved grief during a subsequent pregnancy and dur-ing the postnatal period than parents who have experienced a miscarriage."
5. This is a case report on a young mother with previous stillbirth, experiencing problems at the next birth, which resolve after starting skin-to-skin contact.

Reference List

(1)   Collins S. Baby Stephanie: a case study in compassionate care. Neonatal Intensive Care 1993 March;6(2):47-9.
(2)   Jonas-Simpson C, McMahon E. The Language of Loss When a Baby Dies Prior to Birth: Cocreating Human Experience. Nursing Science Quarterly 2005 April;18(2):124-30.
(3)   Gamble J, Creedy D. Content and Processes of Postpartum Counseling After a Distressing Birth Experience: A Review. Birth: Issues in Perinatal Care 2004 September;31(3):213-8.
(4)   Theut SK, Pedersen FA, Zaslow MJ, Cain RL, Rabinovich BA, Morihisa JM. Perinatal loss and parental bereavement. The American Journal Of Psychiatry 1989 May;146(5):635-9.
(5)   Burkhammer MD, Anderson GC, Sheau-Huey C. Grief, Anxiety, Stillbirth, and Perinatal Problems: Healing With Kangaroo Care. JOGNN: Journal of Obstetric, Gynecologic, & Neonatal Nursing 2004 Novem-ber;33(6):774-82.

RESOURCES

There is a huge amount of information on the internet and in the bookshops, with confusing advice! This is a very small selection of further information that is in line with the information in this manual, and which we recommend. There is a lot more very good information; there is also some which is not so helpful!

DVD / Videos:

By Jill and Nils Bergman:
Restoring the Original Paradigm for infant care and breastfeeding
Rediscover the Natural Way to care for your baby
Hold Your Prem (film version of this book!)
Available at *www.kangaroomothercare.com*
For USA: *www.geddesproduction.com*

By Christina Smillie: *Baby-led Breastfeeding*
By Dr Lennart Righard: *Delivery Self Attachment*
Available at *www.geddesproduction.com*

By Debby Takikawa: *What babies want*

Key websites:

NICU Care

www.kangaroomothercare.com	Skin-to-skin contact
www.prematurity.org	Information on NICU
www.nicuparentsupport.org	NICU parent support
www.compassionatefriends.org	Grief support
http://www.missfoundation.org	When a Child Dies
http://www.missingangelsbill.org	Stillbirth Policy Advocacy

Breastfeeding support

www.breastfeeding.com	
www.lalecheleague.org	
www.ilca.org	
www.hmbana.org	Human Milk Bank Association of North America

Other resources

www.australianbabyhands.com	sign language for babies
www.askdrsears.com	
www.tamba.org.uk	for parents of twins and multiples

Some helpful books to read

The Science of Parenting by Margot Sunderland, 2006. ISBN-13: 978-1-4053-1486-2.

Kangaroo Care: The best you can do to help your preterm infant by Susan Ludington-Hoe, Bantam Books, 1993.

Breastfeeding made simple by Nancy Mohrbacher, 2005. ISBN 1-57224-404-6.

When pregnancy follows a loss by Joann O'Leary. 2006. ISBN-13-978-0-9789439-0-5.

Fathers-to-be handbook by Patrick Houser, available http://fatherstobe.org/

CALMS: a guide to soothing your baby by Carrie Contey, Debby Takikawa http://calmsguide.com/

Come home soon, Baby brother by Debi Iarussi (A colouring in book for siblings of prems)

Sleeping with your baby by James Mc Kenna, Platypus Media.

Bonding by M. Klaus, J Kennell and P.Klaus.

Your amazing newborn by M. Klaus and P. Klaus, Perseus Books.

Why love Matters by Sue Gerhardt, Routledge, Taylor and Francis.

Biological Nurturing: laid-back breastfeeding by Dr Suzanne Colson, available from www.geddesproduction.com

Sweet Dreams: A pediatrician's secrets for your child's good night's sleep by Dr Paul Fleiss, Lowell House, Illinois.

Best medicine: Human milk in the NICU by Drs. Nancy Wight, Jane Morton, and Jai Kim. Hale Publishing.

Gentle Birth, Gentle Mothering by Dr Sarah Buckley, One Moon Press Brisbane Australia.

From the author

Thank you to the many people who have helped to make this book happen:

- the parents of premature babies who shared deeply with me; their experiences will help other parents who now have to walk this road;
- the parents who let us take photos of them and their babies;
- the nurses, doctors, developmental specialists and researchers who are so dedicated to premature babies and their parents;
- Peter Hartmann for permission to use his thermal image on page 51;
- Louise Goosen for letting me use a number of her photographs;
- Hilary Palser for her faithful encouragement in walking me through this book;
- Agneta Kleberg and Welma Lubbe for insights on developmental care;
- Ronel Gabriels for input on grief counselling
- Bronwyn Lusted and Ann Westoby for their diagrams;
- Paddy O'Leary my insightful and patient editor;
- Barbara Mueller for being such an encouragement in typesetting and bringing this book to completion.

My great thanks go to my husband Nils for all of his 20 years of holding onto his vision for improving the start for premature babies. He has distilled this broad-based knowledge from thousands of articles. He has continuously encouraged me to "translate" the medical jargon into everyday English for every parent. What a privilege to have such a wonderful husband, work partner and friend!

Above all, thank you Jesus, for the miracle of life and for being my SAFE place.

CPSIA information can be obtained at www.ICGtesting.com
Printed in the USA
BVOW03s0843260216

437891BV00005B/26/P

9 781920 411336